CHARM YOUR CLIENTS

Neuromarketing for Vets

Inmaculada Pérez Madrigal
Miguel Ángel Valera
Núria Tabares Rivero

Plaza Antonio Beltrán Martínez nº 1, planta 8 - letra I
(Centro empresarial El Trovador)
50002 Zaragoza - Spain

First printing: January 2019

This book was originally published in Spanish under the title:
Enamora a tu cliente. Neuromarketing *para veterinarios*
© 2018 Grupo Asís Biomedia, SL
ISBN Spanish edition: 978-84-17225-49-0

Translation:
Neil Ashby

Illustrator:
Israel Hernández Rubio

ISBN: 978-84-17640-03-3
DL: Z 1556-2018

Design, layout and printing:
Servet editorial - Grupo Asís Biomedia, SL
www.grupoasis.com
info@grupoasis.com

Servet is the publishing house of Grupo Asís

Warning:

Veterinary science is constantly evolving, as are pharmacology and the other sciences. Inevitably, it is therefore the responsibility of the veterinary surgeon to determine and verify the dosage, the method of administration, the duration of treatment and any possible contraindications to the treatments given to each individual patient, based on his or her professional experience. Neither the publisher nor the author can be held liable for any damage or harm caused to people, animals or properties resulting from the correct or incorrect application of the information contained in this book.

ACKNOWLEDGEMENTS

Dear reader,

Firstly, thank you for your curiosity and interest in turning your veterinary clinic into a place where you can work in harmony with your team, your clients, and your patients. All of you will benefit from that curiosity and interest when you start applying neuromarketing techniques.

Let me tell you how this work came into being.

When I suggested to Inma Pérez that we write this book together, I knew she wouldn't be able to say no. I first met Inma when I helped her implement health plans for her clinic. The weekend was a mixture of work and pleasure, because I was with my family and because we became friends. In fact, she had been thinking about writing a book for some time but needed an encouraging nudge. Inma is an expert in nonverbal communication and neuromarketing, so I couldn't pass up on the opportunity.

As luck would have it, a few days after committing to the project she mentioned it to her colleague Núria Tabares. She described the project with so much enthusiasm that Núria asked if she could also participate; now it was me who couldn't say no. Núria is a certified coach and very familiar with the tools needed to make teams grow and achieve their goals together.

Anyone who has written a book is aware of the work involved, not just writing it, but the planning, revision, constant communication with the publisher, and so on. When three different authors are involved, the search for a common language complicates the task, although it usually results in a more polished final product as each chapter is reviewed by all three collaborators, regardless of who wrote it. You cannot imagine how pernickety we can be with each other's work to ensure the text is unsurpassable. Therefore, I would like to thank Inma and Núria for their patience and self-imposed standards of excellence.

I sincerely hope, dear reader, that you discover lots of answers to questions about neuromarketing and can create the best real and virtual spaces to develop your business further and, most importantly, that you spend many happy hours in your clinic.

Mike Valera

THE AUTHORS

Inmaculada Pérez Madrigal

Inmaculada graduated in veterinary medicine and holds an MBA; she has managed the Plaza de España veterinary clinic in Cádiz for the past 12 years (www.clinicaveterinariacadiz.com).

She works in customer service and management, in combination with her duties as a primary care veterinary practitioner. Inma provides consultancy and training seminars on sales techniques for veterinary surgeons. During 2015, she contributed to the bimonthly publication Canis et Felis with articles on neuromarketing.

She is currently a member of the Spanish Small Animal Veterinary Association (AVEPA), the Spanish Association of Veterinary Clinic Management (AGESVET), the Madrid Small Animal Veterinary Association (AMVAC), and the Cádiz Business Association of Veterinary Clinics (AEVECCA).

Miguel Ángel Valera

A veterinary surgeon since 1990, Miguel Ángel started to offer health plans to his clients at Centauro Veterinarios in 1993 (www.centauroveterinarios.com).

Drawing upon his more than 20 years of experience with plans as his main working instrument, he created Plans4Vets to provide clinics with advice on designing health plans and developing skills in basic sales and marketing techniques (www.mascotasyplanes.com). In 2017, his book *Planes de Salud* (*Health Plans*) was published by Editorial Servet.

He spends his spare time singing with the group MUSIC STOP (www.musicstop.es).

Núria Tabares Rivero

Núria graduated in veterinary medicine (Autonomous University of Barcelona) and holds a postgraduate diploma in executive and career coaching (University of Barcelona). She regularly gives lectures on relational communication, conflict management, teamwork and marketing.

She sat for ten years on the Veterinary Practice Standards Committee of the College of Veterinary Surgeons of Barcelona and is a former president of Agesvet (Spanish Association of Veterinary Surgeons Specialised in Veterinary Practice Management). From 2001 to 2018 she was co-owner of the company C.V. Manescal S.c.p., which incorporates the Manescalia Veterinaris clinic.

She currently owns the company Coaching Ability (www.coachingability.com).

PREFACE

What motivates people to buy things? What tools can we use to persuade a client to acquire our services?

Vets generally lack training in marketing and sales. Graduate degrees do not teach us how to sell our work. Neuromarketing is a great resource when trying to understand what motivates your clients to purchase services, so you can work on earning their loyalty throughout the process and developing skills to ensure they fall in love with your clinic.

If you know how the client's mind works, it is much easier to offer the services their pet needs with honesty, ethically and for the benefit of both the owner and their pet.

That is why we recommend you implement neuromarketing coherently across all levels of your veterinary clinic. Using appropriate language and creating a favourable environment can encourage the client to select the best option for their pet.

In this book, the authors offer their experience gleaned from over 20 years working in different areas of veterinary practice. It is a practical manual that combines up-to-date knowledge about neuromarketing with practical ideas for implementing this know-how in the real-world routine of any veterinary clinic. *Charm Your Clients. Neuromarketing for Vets* is suitable for both small clinics and larger centres that wish to improve their sales techniques.

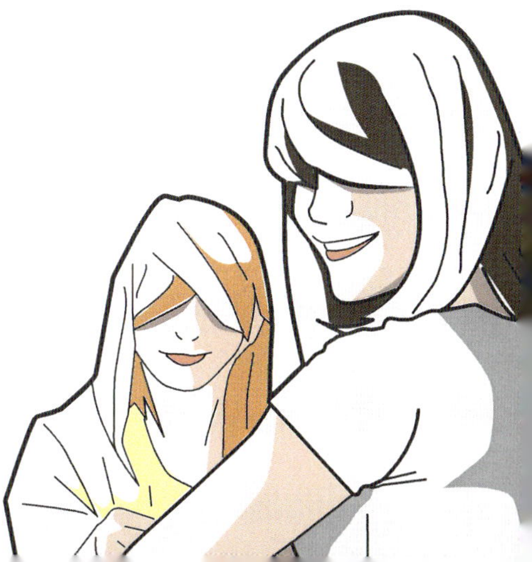

FOREWORD

"They didn't say anything about this in the [medical] books"... is the first line of *All Creatures Great and Small* by James Herriot, which describes the trials and tribulations of a country vet based on the author's real-life experiences.

Veterinary medicine has changed dramatically since those bygone years in which Herriot narrated his stories, back in the 1930s, 40s, and 50s. This evolution has touched all aspects of veterinary practice, ranging from professional training methods to the most complex of specialisations currently being exercised, and including diagnostic tools, surgical techniques, and major advances in the prevention and treatment of diseases.

A predominant aspect of these industry-wide developments, especially when it comes to pets, is the transformation involving those who use our services, in other words, our clients. There is a now wide range of products and services for pets; we are surrounded by pet-friendly venues, and witness to an increasingly common and extra special bond between families and their cats and dogs. Rather than criticising or judging this level of relationship, those of us working in the sector must learn to understand it so we can adapt to it effectively for the benefit of everyone involved.

As in Herriot's day, the medical books do not allude to these extraclinical considerations (and to be honest, they shouldn't have to). Fortunately, this evolution has also led to the publication of books like this one. This work presents the material needed to address concerns that are increasingly worthy of our attention, such as: an understanding of the client's emotions and what drives them to select a veterinary clinic; how to develop skills so we may effectively promote the measures required to keep pets healthier; the design of services that generate satisfaction in our patients' owners and help us gain their loyalty; and how to form harmonious and productive work teams. This is where neuromarketing comes in, since it can help us decipher the behavioural "whims" of our clients and coworkers, and use them to the everyone's benefit.

Charm Your Clients. Neuromarketing for Vets provides a very warm welcome to this world, a world that is essential for anyone who wishes to develop all facets of their professional growth.

You will find it very useful, and I am sure you will enjoy it.

Alex Grassie
DVM Mercadotecnia
CIMA veterinary centre, Mexico

I feel honoured that the authors Inmaculada Pérez, Núria Tabares, and Miguel Ángel Valera have asked me to write a brief introduction to their book *Charm Your Clients. Neuromarketing for Vets*. I have known each of them for years, since we worked together on various veterinary management projects and forums, where they always stood out because of their professional commitment, creativity, and constant search for excellence. They have collectively accumulated extensive experience as veterinary practice owners and managers (all three of them), as an executive and career coach (Núria), as a designer of and consultant in health plans (Miguel Ángel), and as an author and instructor in veterinary sales techniques (Inmaculada).

Simply being a competent veterinary professional is not enough in our highly demanding vocation; we need to understand our clients, and how and why they make their decisions. We also manage emotions. Therefore, I can think of at least six reasons why I would recommend this book to any veterinary surgeon who wishes to get more out of the routine aspects of their profession:

1. It is innovative; plenty has been written about neuromarketing and a fair amount about marketing for veterinary clinics, but this is one of the few books that brings together both disciplines.
2. It is both very practical and thorough; the book is based on models that have been tested extensively in neuroscience and social psychology but applies them to very specific situations faced during a vet's routine practice (in the examining room, reception, when preparing estimates, on the telephone, managing health plans, etc.).
3. It is an enjoyable and enlightening read; veterinary surgeons can finally understand the reactions they have so often observed in their clients.
4. It is a profitable book; it teaches you how to offer more attractive and convincing services to your clients, but without having to make any drastic changes to your current routines; you simply need to present them better.
5. It is a contemporary work; the book discusses current tendencies, technology, social media, and essentially the modern client who enters your clinic.
6. The authors are perfectly qualified to write this book as they combine broad clinical experience with training in various fields of business and a lively intellectual curiosity that has driven them to collaborate in diverse projects throughout their careers.

Pere Mercader

Founding partner of Veterinary Management Studies

Veterinary clinician

INTRODUCTION

Throughout the 20th century, veterinary clinics grew in an amicable business environment thanks to a low level of competition. However, since the turn of the century, the arrival of new forms of business, an increasing number of professionals, and the low profitability and significant financial pressure in our sector have forced us to learn how to maximise profit in our businesses.

The development of neuromarketing techniques designed to sell services is a hot topic in all markets, but, until now, there weren't any texts, besides a few articles, adapted to meet the needs of veterinary clinics.

What is more, the word sales has always been a taboo or an Achilles heel for veterinary practices. Vets diagnose and treat animals, we don't like to sell things. However, if you don't earn the owner's trust, you cannot provide everything that the patient needs. That is what neuromarketing is all about, earning client loyalty, knowing how to gain their trust, and ensuring you are in their thoughts every time they look at their pet. The aim is to produce a partnership, a sincere relationship with your client.

We now know how to win our clients' trust and what they value in a professional, and we have put these techniques into practice; therefore, we have decided to divulge this information in this practical book for veterinary surgeons.

We spend a lot of time training and studying to become vets; we have inquisitive minds and need to be given a lot of reasons before changing how we do things. Nevertheless, we forget that purchasing decisions, or factors such as trust, are based on emotions rather than rationale, which is where neuromarketing comes in. Our failed attempts to win over clients are sometimes down to misguided communication or a lack of familiarity about how we should present our work. It is as simple and as pitiful as that.

The aim of this book is to explain how our clients see us, how they perceive us, and what we must do to improve our communication with them and our team by applying the same techniques employed in large companies. We need to learn how to offer our services to gain the client's trust and differentiate ourselves from other clinics. That is why we talk about using neuromarketing to communicate with the client, our work colleagues and collaborators, and when designing our clinics.

The book starts with a brief description of the areas of the brain and decision-making processes. It then analyses market trends in the fields of human and veterinary medicine. We continue by explaining how to use different communication techniques in the clinic, how to give an estimate for some work, and a basic subject – telephone skills. You will also find information about how to present your business from a neuromarketing perspective and, finally, we discuss staff and how to improve internal communication. The book ends with some exercises designed to help the reader put into practice what they have learnt.

They say a salesperson is born, not made; but we can learn to do anything, and techniques for selling services or better communication skills are no exception. It is just a question of desire and a willingness to do things differently.

TABLE OF CONTENTS

1 What is neuromarketing and how can it be used?

Why write a book about neuromarketing for veterinary clinicians?

Veterinary clinics are more than just companies, they are emotional businesses based on the bond people establish with their pets. Our clinics are going through a process of rapid evolution in line with current social changes that have altered how we perceive animals. A clear example is how people's relationship with their pets has developed over the years; decades ago, animals were regarded as merely another piece of work equipment, but now they have become our new fur babies.

Neuromarketing explains sale processes from an emotional perspective.

It is often said that a nation can be judged by the way it treats its animals, and in recent years all businesses in the pet sector have enjoyed continuous growth, whether they deal with food, aesthetics, training, or health services.

The rise of social media has meant that some of our clients have lost their connection with fee-based services, such as those offered by veterinary surgeons, as they now look for the same services and advice online, where they are often considerably cheaper or even free.

Hence, we must create and reinforce our clients' emotional bond with their veterinary practice, and neuromarketing works from this perspective.

Neuromarketing is a fusion between marketing and neuroscience. It offers companies the opportunity to work on elements such as customer loyalty, customer service, corporate image, and the generation of pleasure. You can extract profitability from these techniques by implementing them in your veterinary centre after analysing what clients really want, what is important to them, and the qualities they value in their vet. That is why neuromarketing adapts so well to our type of business and you can use it to study consumers and how they consume.

In the 21st century, we are witnessing ever-faster changes, as well as job losses because companies are developing more efficient internal processes that require less workers. However, given that vets belong to the services sector, our businesses will survive because machines are yet to be created that can diagnose complex diseases, palpate, or perform parenteral drug administration.

Our competitive edge as veterinary practitioners is that we are essential for maintaining our clients' pets in good health. Neuromarketing helps us emphasise this point to our clients.

Emotions originate in the primitive brain, in the depth of our being. Nevertheless, minimally invasive, real-time diagnostic imaging techniques have opened a window into the consumer's mind and shed light on methods to ensure we make a sale and our estimates are accepted.

We have traditionally tended to believe that good salespeople and communicators are born with a gift. Despite this, neuromarketing shows we can measure the impact different images, sounds, and phrases have on the brain, and learn to employ techniques that will help us attain more successful outcomes. Good salespeople have always used these techniques, albeit intuitively, but now we know why certain people succeed where others fail.

We shall also examine the method, so you can offer your clients everything they need using the correct means, learn how to adapt your marketing to your ideal clients, and become familiar with client loyalty-building and retention mechanisms. As managers and professionals, you must improve your communication techniques to reach your clients and employees, while learning how to engage the latter in sales processes.

Some basic theory

Neuromarketing is based on the use of neuroscientific methods to analyse and understand human behaviour and emotions with respect to the market and trading.

In the 1960s, companies became interested in discovering why people select one product over another. They started to conduct surveys and launch products with new flavours, or the same ones but packaged differently. They noticed that consumers often lie, as products that were successful in prelaunch trials later failed when released on the real market.

These failures led to the creation of more sophisticated questions and means of measuring responses. After the questionnaires came the round-table debates, and then the use of complicated helmets to scan different areas of the brain. We now have technology that can measure, in real-time, which areas of the brain "light up" when they are shown a product or experience an emotion. Combining scientific knowledge from sociologists, pedagogues, and neurologists, marketing specialists analyse people's responses to different types of stimulation and can even study the variation in responses from healthy and diseased brains.

It had long been considered that one side of the brain was responsible for rational processes and the other for emotional ones. Purchasing decisions were thought to be rational choices; we made comparisons and selections based on measured and objective patterns. However, alternative experiments have shown that the brain does not always follow logic, it makes misleading decisions in certain situations. Therefore, the brain does not always make rational decisions.

Sales techniques

Can you use these techniques in small companies? Are they suitable for vets? Which processes are involved?

These techniques were first applied according to basic trial and error methods; they were implemented and rated as successful or otherwise. In our case, clients visited our clinics with fixed budgets to spend on their pet's surgery. For years, we practiced with neuromarketing methods to provide estimates that increased the range of services offered, such as complementary laboratory tests or inpatient services.

A fusion of marketing and neuroscience

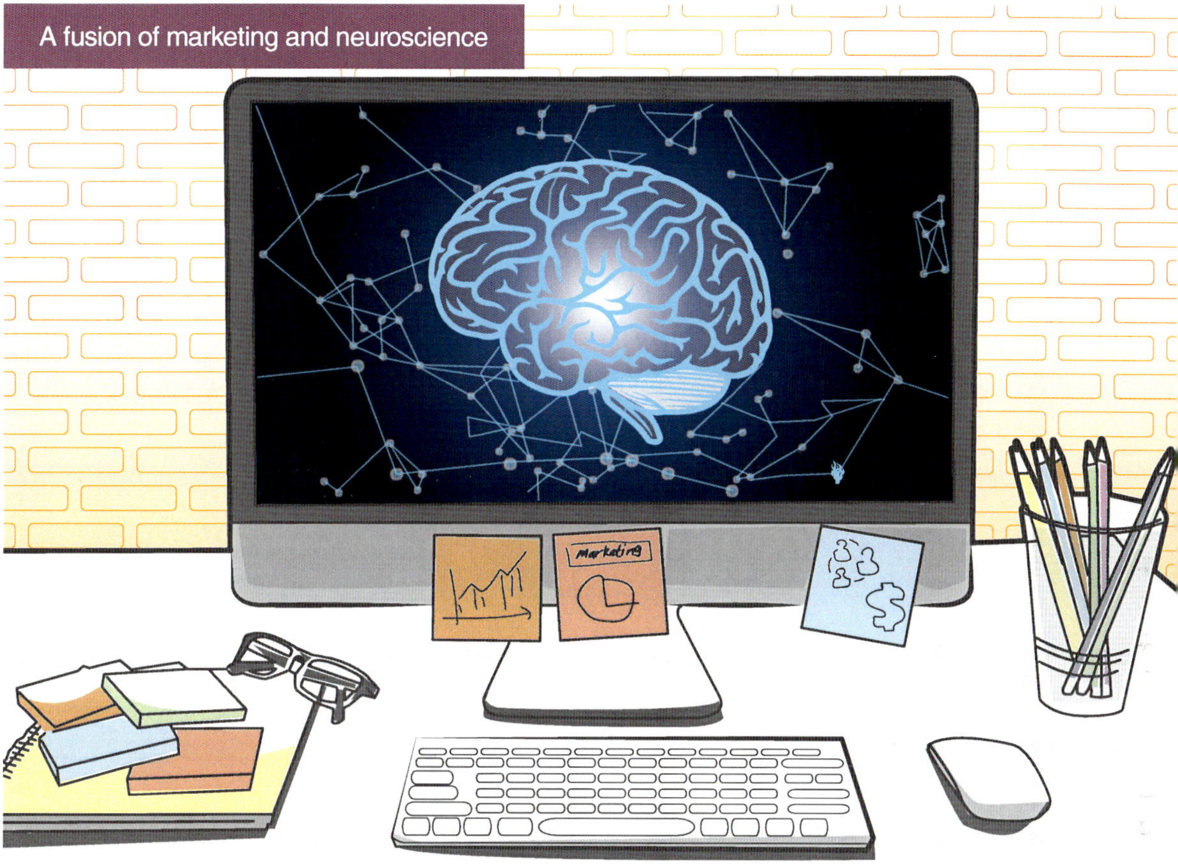

To our surprise we found that these methods worked very well in our practice. We then asked ourselves whether these techniques could be exported or if the methods only work after experiencing a learning curve.

We started to apply neuromarketing by changing how we answered the telephone. There was a genuine impact on revenue, so we continued working along the same lines. Later we installed two new telephone lines because clients find it very frustrating when they must ring several times to make an appointment.

There are no magic tricks, formulae for success, sales buttons, or specific techniques that produce miraculous results; neuromarketing is a multifactor technique. However, the use of various coherent tools, which do not alarm the consumer, will swing the balance in your favour at just the right moment.

TIP

Before trying to implant any methods, it is a good idea to analyse where you are, what type of clinic you have now and want to have in the future, and whether your model is coherent.

Let us start with a straightforward example. Within a few seconds of entering a restaurant and taking in the decoration and staff's attire, you can guess the final bill for a meal without looking at the menu. If wood predominates throughout the avant-garde decor, the dining rooms are large and well-lit, and every detail has been considered, from the table linen and dinnerware to staff service, you can assume that it will cost a lot more than the lunchtime menu at the local café.

However, you will still praise the exceptional service of each eatery if they both exceed your expectations, even though these expectations may differ widely for the two premises. This is known as experiential neuromarketing.

You must seek the same coherence and avoid confusing the consumer in your clinic. These points are very important when setting the price for services and you should use the same tools to earn customer loyalty as those employed by large companies:

- Work on the key points.
- Exceed expectations.
- Make clients feel they belong to a special group.
- Reward loyalty.

The aim is to ensure pet owners perceive added value in every clinical procedure or visit to the centre, so that your clinic is always the first choice that comes to mind.

2 Integrity and beliefs. Ethics in neuromarketing

The application of neuromarketing leads us to ask ourselves whether it is ethical to use our knowledge of the human mind for sales purposes.

Large companies encourage unnecessary consumption, resulting in the appearance of new psychological disorders such as consumer addiction and compulsive shopping. It is also known that purchasing patterns start to be established in children as young as 3 years old. Therefore, advertising generally targets child audiences (particularly in shopping centres, which try to form a connection between consumption and leisure from very early ages) to such an extent that, as consumers, we could question our freedom of choice in light of so many influences.

Increasingly sophisticated sales methods are being deployed. Hence it is important we are familiar with them, not just from a business perspective, but so that we can defend ourselves as consumers by learning to recognise how and when we are being enticed to consume. We must teach future generations how to purchase and control their budget. Knowledge of these methods means we are less susceptible to manipulation.

However, we are not fitted with an on/off switch for shopping and there are no magic wands that can turn consumers into zombies. Nevertheless, there is a combination of techniques that can lead to a successful sale if you manage to give the consumer what they want. We use the word "want" deliberately, because it is not a matter of what the consumer needs; currently, most purchases in the developed world are not due to necessity, but rather because of desire or for pleasure. We live in a hedonistic world and must structure our entire sales strategy around this premise.

We should also remember that we are, above all, veterinary surgeons: our aim is to provide our patients with the best medical attention at any given moment. Yet we must go through an intermediary, namely the animal's owner, who is also the one paying the bill. Therefore, neuromarketing focuses on the owner. You need to ensure the client perceives the vet as an ally who is there to look after their pet's welfare. Estimates are more readily accepted once you have established trust-based relationships. This will result in healthier, more profitable companies, higher levels of client satisfaction, and greater protection for their pets.

TIP

Never recommend anything the animal does not need or make decisions (from a paternalistic perspective) for the owner in order to close a sale, because an aggressive sales technique could result in more complaints.

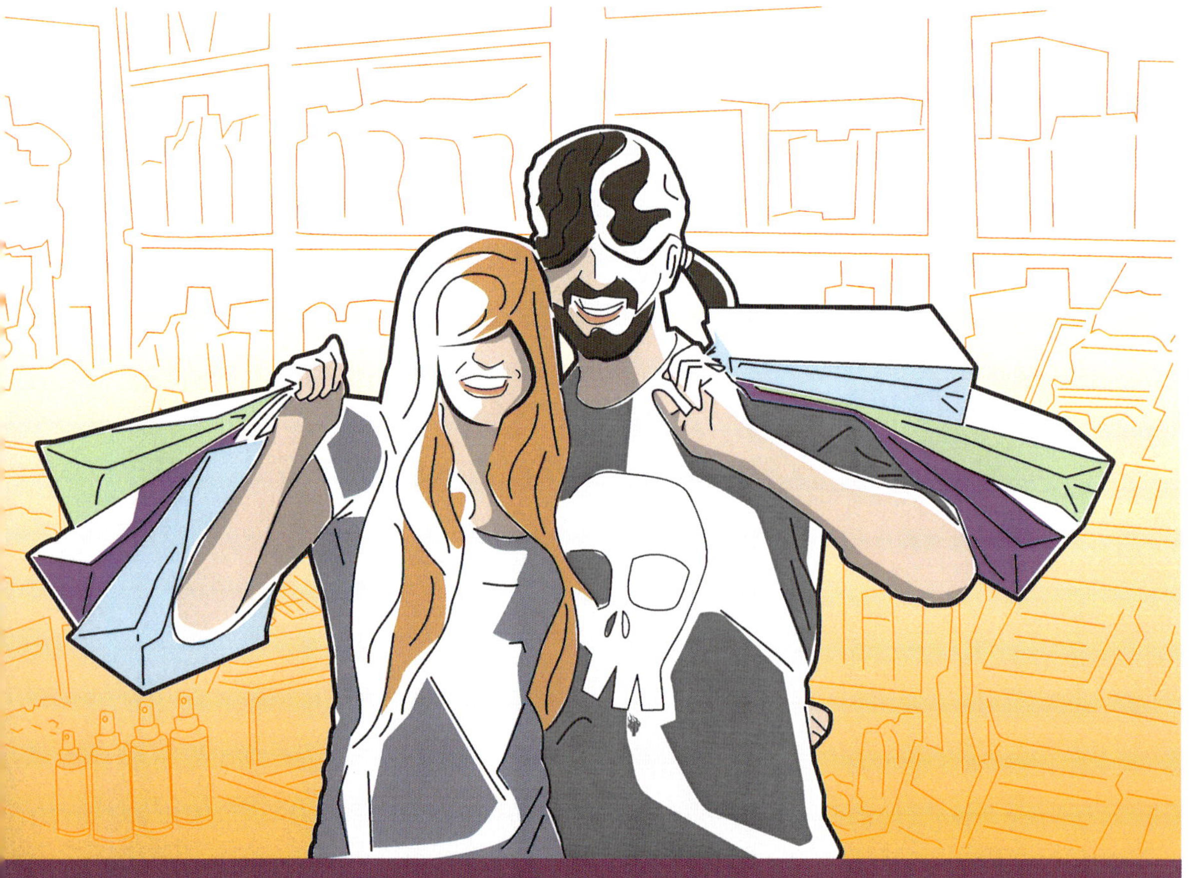

Shopping for pleasure

Pressurising the client may curb their future purchasing, whereas gaining their loyalty is essential for the business. The dissatisfaction of clients who were subject to pressure could lead to a bad press and affect your reputation as a vet. Word-of-mouth is still the best means of attracting new clients.

In human medicine, there are less complaints when patients or their relatives feel the medical team has done everything within their power and were proactively involved in the patient's care. As we humans are social beings, we need to believe our suffering is understood by others.

The fear and stress owners experience during a consultation can inhibit their decision-making process. You must help clients select the most appropriate treatment option in each case. However, if the owner feels they have not chosen freely, but rather they were forced into a decision, and the animal gets worse and dies, they will lay the blame on the veterinary surgeon. The vet and owner must reach mutual decisions as partners who seek the best for the patient.

You must also avoid manipulating clients through fear, but instead act with consistency and integrity, which means you should never prescribe unnecessary medications or recommend needless diagnostic tests. Having said that, by contrast you should prescribe everything required to improve the patient's health, focusing on a solution to the owner's current problem.

The limits of neuromarketing are yet to be defined because it is a relatively young science and it remains unclear how much we can achieve by combining our knowledge of the brain and behaviour together with progressively more sophisticated advertising and sales techniques. It is true that increasingly targeted sales methods are being employed, and we still do not know to what extent we are susceptible. Every year, there are more and more cases of disorders such as compulsive shopping and consumer addiction. The use of cards and the rise of new payment methods that eliminate the need for cash as a tangible item only add to these problems.

Maybe legal regulations will be developed in the future to protect consumers and restrict advertising, but until then learning to identify the marketing techniques we are exposed to could protect us from making purchases and investments in our businesses that are based on emotion instead of reasoning.

3 What makes people buy things?

What drives us to consume? Do emotions influence the purchasing process? Why do our clients use veterinary services? To answer these and other questions we need to understand how the human control centre, that is, the brain, works.

Anatomy of the decision-making brain

The brain is a unique organ that has developed over millions of years. It was not designed in a single step, rather it is the product of an evolutionary process. Nevertheless, only a short time has passed in evolutionary terms and, in a way, we are still Cro-Magnons.

During any experience, for example, when contemplating the landscape, the brain processes, compiles, and filters an array of input to give us an image of our surroundings. It also creates different types of memory depending on the experience.

Compared to other animals, the human brain is neither the largest nor the most intricate. Curiously, it also shrinks as we get older. What differentiates humans from other living beings and endows us with cognitive advantages is our larger and more complicated association cortex. For example, the human neocortex differs greatly from that of a rat; it is much larger than the proportionally tiny rat neocortex which has not developed the same functions as in primates. Therefore, the consequences of damage to a rat's neocortex are insignificant, but a person may be unable to walk if they were to suffer a similar injury.

The brain's negative growth with age is somewhat paradoxical, as it is the only organ that grows smaller as we get older while its capacity simultaneously increases. Furthermore, huge numbers of neurons die before the age of 7 years, particularly in the first 3 years of childhood. Neural circuits are established and reinforced by eliminating neurons, so the ones that are not used die. This is how the brain adapts to the environment in which it is born. These neural networks are unique to each brain, which gives rise to individuals with specific talents compared to others with different skills.

For our present purposes we need to introduce the parts of the brain, but we shall not describe its anatomy in detail. However, we must provide a basic classification of the different areas and functions to continue discussing the decision-making process.

The brain is divided into two hemispheres, left and right, interconnected by the corpus callosum. In a broad simplification, we can state that each side of the brain processes information differently in most people:

- The **left hemisphere** is better at processing language, logic, numbers, sequences, functions, mathematics, and planning. It is more rational and intelligence tests measure the capacity of this hemisphere.
- The **right hemisphere** specialises in the interpretation of images, music, colours, and behaviour, and it processes things more quickly. It provides an overall analysis of situations, combining verbal and auditory information before transmitting it as a complete picture, so we say it is responsible for holistic thinking. It focuses on providing an immediate response.

In terms of how it functions, the brain can be divided into three structures at different depths:

- **Lower brain**. Also known as the primitive or reptilian brain, this section functions automatically and subconsciously, and is responsible for decision-making processes. It is like a reptile's brain, hence the name, and is the first portion of brain to grow in human foetuses in the womb. The lower brain is fully developed at around 24 years. It makes basic take-it-or-leave-it type survival decisions. The medulla oblongata automatically or subconsciously controls parameters such as temperature and respiration. Although it is responsible for most decisions we make, the primitive brain shares information with the other structures, so the decision can be justified.
- **Mesencephalon or midbrain**. It senses and processes emotions and feelings. This area of the brain includes control centres, such as the hypothalamus and cerebellum, which govern biological rhythms, and motor and sensory coordination, respectively.
- **Cortex**. This is the brain's outermost layer and the last to develop. It processes rational, conscious information and shares its conclusions with the two deeper structures. It is the only brain structure capable of producing language.

Vomiting and cough centres are located in specific areas of the brain. Meanwhile, memories, which are accumulated or processed in more complicated areas, are transferred between locations. They are initially stored near the hippocampus for a couple of years, but they are later moved to other areas of the cortex.

How do we decide?

Functional magnetic resonance imaging (fMRI) studies have shown that decisions are made emotionally and then justified rationally.

Around 85 % of our decisions are subconscious. Regardless of the decision in hand (whether about clothes, drinks, cars, getting married, etc.) most decisions are subconscious, in fact some experts cite a level of 95 %.

We know that the reptilian brain decides, then the rational brain justifies this decision. When the reptilian brain makes a decision, it actually processes it and mixes it with emotions before passing it to the cortex where this verdict is justified.

Parts of the brain

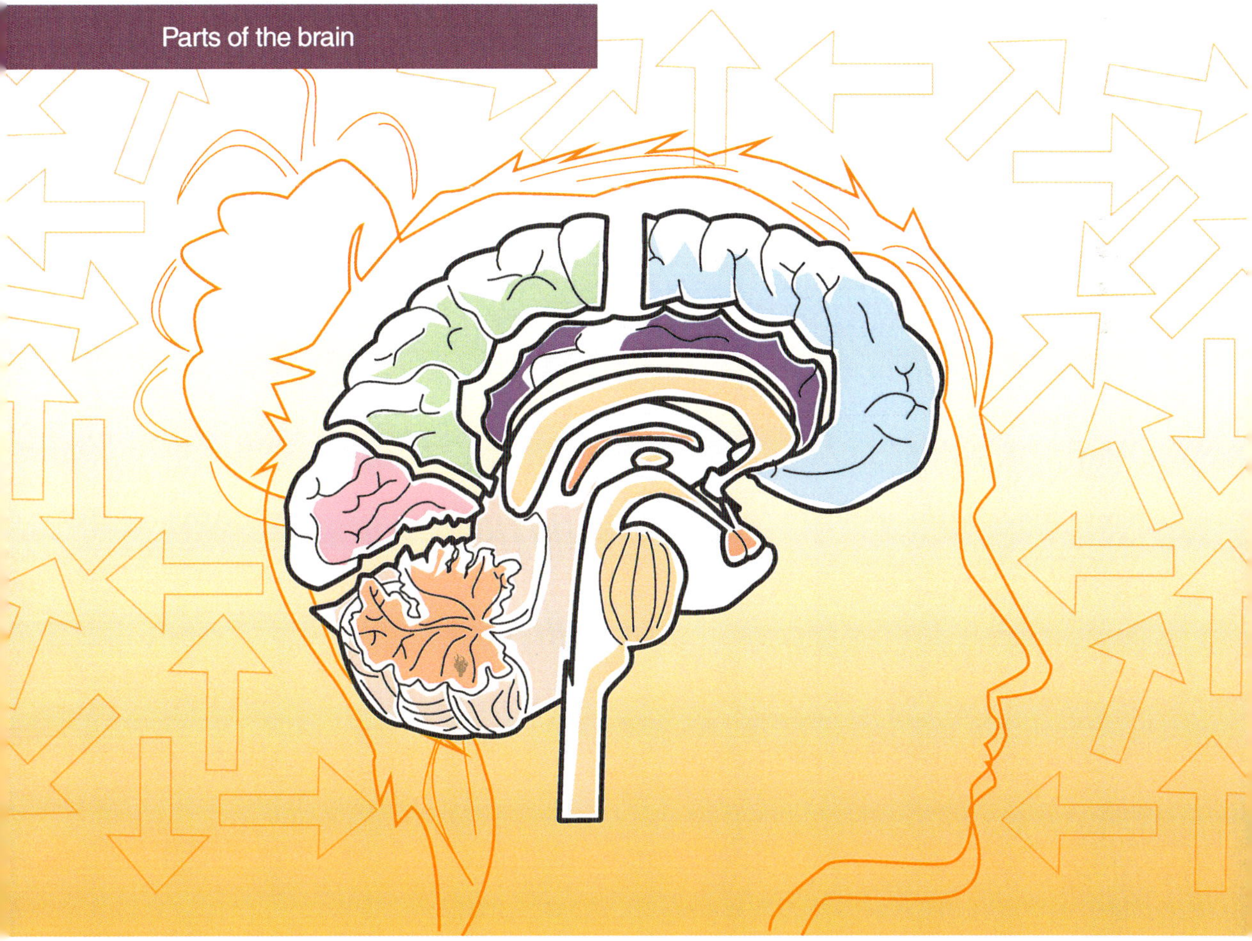

EXAMPLE

The internal dialogue when buying a car would be something like this: I am going to buy this car (it is elegant, wonderful, it would make me feel alive) → really it is an investment → besides, I will use it to go on more weekend trips (justification). All of which is accompanied by mental images and stories.

What makes people buy things? The role of emotions

When someone purchases a product and they are asked why they made their choice, each person gives their own reasons. However, we know that these are not the true reasons for their choice. People lie in questionnaires.

Maybe you had no intention of buying anything while walking down the street, but an open door entices you into a shop. Then you spot a jumper that reminds you of the one your mother knitted when you were young, and you buy it arguing that you like the colour. Although you do not realise, this is not the true reason behind your purchase.

Why choose one colour over another? We do not know why a given person likes, for example, the colour yellow, maybe because it elicits a memory. Yet we do know that emotions affect every single decision we make.

Emotions are adaptive processes that prioritise situations and help people achieve their objectives. They help us decide in difficult situations. Emotions can modify our actions by acting as switches that adjust our behaviour, and they are also involved in the memory process. Each one is associated with a facial expression that we must learn to recognise. This is where mirror neurons come in, but these will be discussed later.

In the sales process, besides emotions we must also consider previous experiences, personal stories, and how people feel when faced with the given situation. These past experiences create a short- or long-term memory depending on the intensity of the event.

Each emotion can be linked to a specific facial expression. The basic ones are: fear, happiness, sadness, surprise, and disgust. Others to consider are: greed, shame, boredom, love, insecurity, and elevation.

Pleasure, gratitude, pride, interest, and elevation are very important in sales. Elevation is a sense of belonging to something greater and engagement with one's surroundings.

REASONS WHY WE CONSUME

1. An attempt at avoiding fear; the act of consuming is associated with security. Fear of disease makes us invest in healthcare or high-quality food products. Fear of shortage make us invest in property.
2. Humans are gatherers, we now gather from shops. Touching or smelling items before buying them appears to be related to the purchasing process.
3. The primitive brain seeks a sense of power, security, and strength. Therefore, it looks for large objects and associates size with quality or power. Driving a large, eye-catching car makes one feel successful and manufacturers exploit this element.
4. Affiliation with a certain group or class also affects the purchasing process. Humans are social beings and we want to be accepted by the group or belong to a select elite. Identification with the group's values creates a strong emotional link with the mark. Examples of belonging are owning a Harley-Davidson, or several pets, living and consuming ecologically, or wearing designer labels.
5. Showing our strength places us on the top rungs of the evolutionary, and reproductive, ladder. Consumption is the opportunity to showcase success...

The main emotional factors that bear an influence on consumption are:

- **Fear.** This is one of the most primitive feelings and is associated with the amygdala. There are many types of fear, for example fear of physical pain, but two the most significant types are fear of uncertainty and fear of ridicule. In fact, these are very primitive and torment humans more than any others. Fear impedes and paralyses, it leads to a mental state that inhibits decision-making and stops us from taking risks. If we manage to block out this fear, for example through creative thinking or by emphasising positive information, this facilitates the decision-making process by extracting the person from their paralysis. Anxiety is also known to increase fear, so we want to quell this feeling. Ambiguities also block the decision-making brain because we are faced with the unknown.
- **Pleasure**. This is the opposite of pain, it is extreme happiness, and sometimes we must decide between obtaining immediate pleasure or delaying it until later. For example, the choice could lie between spending some money now on a pair of shoes or saving it towards a holiday in the future. Nevertheless, we could choose the option of buying now with a credit card (immediate pleasure) and paying later, thus postponing the pain related to the loss of money. Pleasure is connected to the act of purchasing, the desire, and the sense of ownership, which minimise anxiety and fear.

Why do our clients buy our services?

In the context of a veterinary consultation, there are various reasons:

- Clients consume because they can. The standard of living has increased in the last 30 years, which has had a positive effect on our market. Families are smaller and have greater resources available to them than 30 years ago.
- The connection with and humanisation of pets is a global phenomenon; they are viewed as another member of the family. They are dressed, wrapped up, fed, and cared for as if they were babies. Owners identify with their animals and want to give them the same healthy, natural diet as they seek for themselves. That is why some shops and clinics offer a range of green superfoods.

At the same time there is also a demand for high-quality medical services. A similarity between human and veterinary medicine has been established in the client's mind.

- Neoteny or the puppy principle. Our brains connect with everything that has big eyes and a large forehead. Neoteny makes people treat dogs like babies and their tendency to have large eyes and broad foreheads causes us to establish bonds with our animals to the extent that we speak to and cuddle them.

Even in their absence, a photo of a puppy always arouses an "aww". The trend for chondrodystrophic breeds relates to the neoteny principle; you only need to look at the face of a Bulldog to notice how huggable they are.

- The sense of belonging to a special group. Expressions such as, "to own a dog, you must be able to look after it well, and I can afford it" would fall within this group. Owning and loving an animal makes pet owners feel special, more sensitive, and better people. They have Facebook groups and websites for their pets. They interact on social networks more than other groups and search for all kinds of information, although not always from vets.
- Fear of death and disease. These factors increase the consumption of medical products and related services, such as health plans or insurance. People consume to feel secure and avoid fear. Remember that fear creates a long-term memory. It is very important that you know how to handle fear during a veterinary appointment. As vets we can come across a range of scenarios:
  1. A client who has experienced the current disease in a previous pet. This can make the appointment unpleasant for the client.
  2. One of the reasons why clients change between vets is because they lost a pet in a given clinic and still suffer from grief; therefore, they change centres when they get a new pet to avoid facing this negative memory. Learning how to handle these situations is very important.
  3. Fear of the unknown. As pets cannot talk, the owner does not know what is wrong with them. Uncertainty creates anxiety, which in turn increases fear. Remember that fear causes paralysis and the owner needs a professional to help them decide what to do. Someone who is afraid, anxious, or panic-stricken can freeze up and find it hard to concentrate or decide. You must learn to handle these emotional states in your clients.
- The owner's search for security as a mechanism to escape pain means the vet needs to relate to the client differently, because they now require another kind of attention. Factors such as opening times, additional services, or veterinary experience can persuade the client to choose one practice over another.

One can and must take advantage of what the market currently has to offer. It is true that competitive pressure has grown in the last 30 years; however, our sociocultural level has also benefited from parallel development. The key to success is learning how to establish trust-based relationships with your clients that can make you stand out from the rest, so mentally they identify you as being their family vet. Establishing emotional bonds is essential.

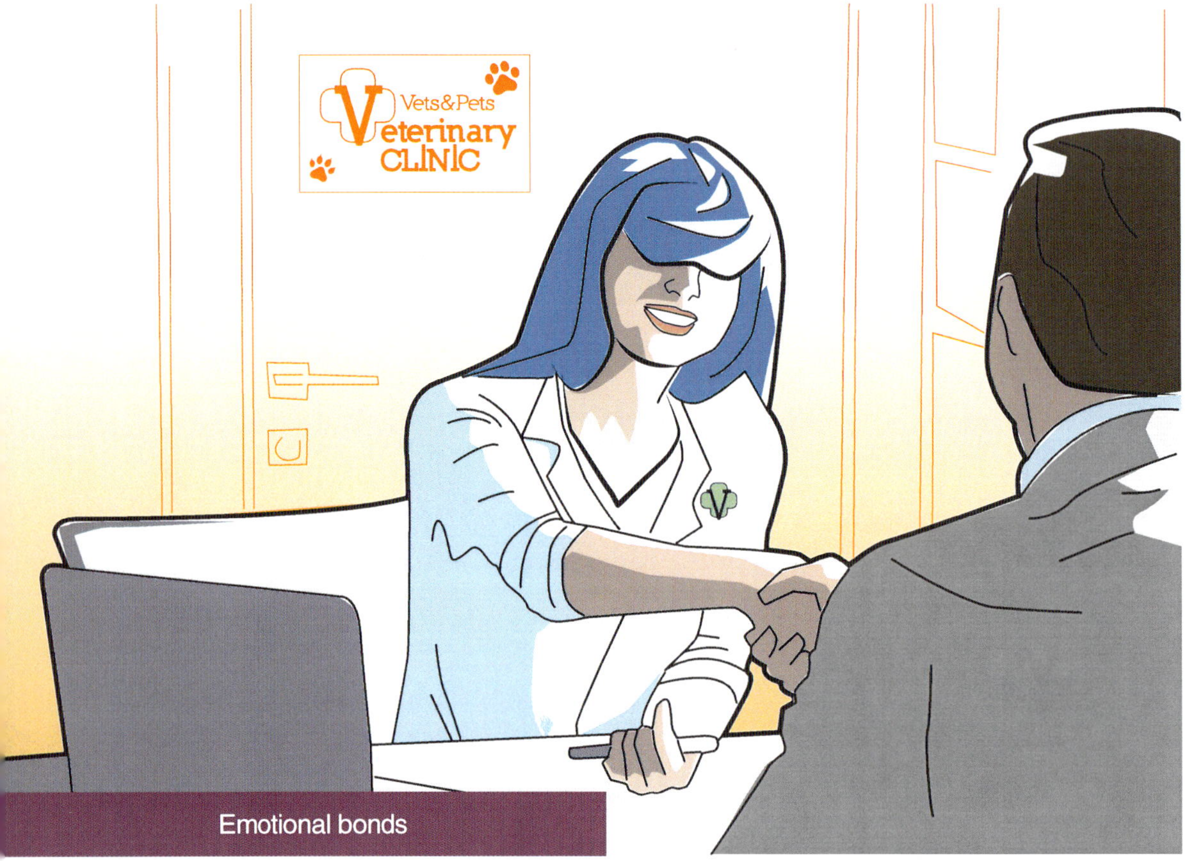

Emotional bonds

4 Future trends in veterinary medicine

The great thing about the 21st century is everything appears to have been decided already, including the future. If we could see it, surely we would do things differently. Nevertheless, there are several studies about trends and sociology which, while they cannot predict exactly where we will be, can offer hints and ideas about the direction the veterinary sector will take over this century. We believe general veterinary medicine is a few years behind human medicine in terms of technical resources, but the tendencies are the same. The future of human medicine is geriatrics, and this will soon be true for veterinary clinics too.

New client profiles

1. Chameleon client

There is already talk about chameleon clients. These clients behave differently depending on the purchasing decisions they must make.

We are all capable of acting like chameleons, for example, we may do everything possible to save money on a flight, but on the other hand we eat out in a luxury restaurant. Similarly, we buy basic unbranded products to save money, yet we are happy to pay more for a specific brand of biscuits.

A chameleon client differentiates between items as either basic commodities or those which have added value and therefore a premium price.

Interestingly, we can no longer classify clients into groups, instead each client will have their own price elasticity curve, desires, and requirements.

This means database management will focus on offering individual clients what they need and studying their consumption patterns. For instance, loyalty cards are used to analyse clients' purchasing habits and facilitate work on cross-sales, although this relies on very powerful computing resources. In our sector, you could individualise health plans, for example, and call them tailored health plans.

2. Trendsetter

A very interesting client model is emerging, known as the trendsetter. They are celebrities and opinion-formers contracted by companies, something which already occurs with YouTubers on the internet. The client is at the centre of the decision-making process, so it is becoming essential to establish real-time, online communication with your clients through the constantly emerging profusion of social media platforms. In the future you will need to find trendsetters and offer them special services, so they recommend you to their followers.

Harmony between different business models

1. Low-cost

This model is here to stay, and even though in our market low-cost is still confused with low price, with time this trend will take on a more professional and profitable form.

Low-cost businesses are materialising in all sectors and across the globe, especially since the 2008 economic downturn. The model is based on completing a lot of operations with very small margins, strict control over spending, and outsourcing more specific and professional services. Some chain stores for pets revolve around the low-cost model and simultaneous cross-selling of veterinary services.

2. High-tech or high-value

This is the counteroffer to the previous model. High value is a much more attractive concept because it features a greater residual margin on each operation.

Both trends will polarise the market, leading to a further reduction in margins, so companies will have to merge to increase their margins by reducing structural and operating costs.

This is already happening in a lot of markets and the veterinary sector will be no exception. The same thing will happen to veterinary distribution businesses.

3. Blue oceans

These will be disruptive and hard to copy, but they will set trends in their sector. They are novel business strategies that help a company stand out from the competition.

4. Shopping centres

They represent a current leisure trend and convenient shopping, but they do not create an emotional link with consumers. The strategy consists of retaining the consumer inside the centre for as long as possible, because the longer they are there, the more they spend. They have a high volume of visitors who are therefore potential shoppers (prospects).

5. Small businesses

The main advantage of the local town centre or small business is they can form an emotional bond with the customer. Traditional markets and neighbourhood shops offer a romantic allure and high level of gratification for consumers. However, the tendency is to concentrate in town centres; therefore, these hubs have become open commercial spaces where the idea is to combine the small market sentiment with the range offered by a shopping centre.

6. Mergers

Falling profit margins and increasing competition will force businesses to join forces and undergo partial or total mergers to survive. The equivalent in our sector would be the proliferation of purchasing cooperatives and diagnostic groups.

Health sectors

The studies available in these areas deal with human medicine, although they can easily be extrapolated to the veterinary sector.

In this segment, the consumer needs to know more. Therefore, a great business opportunity will be large hospitals with well-developed patient communication and connection techniques. The connection will be influenced by the human factor as well as aspects such as internal design and structure. This means that the centre's appearance, the design of waiting rooms, uniforms, etc., will be very important, as will the use of information technology to stay in contact with clients.

An emerging market in human medicine is the demand for luxury health services, so the same thing is predicted to occur in the veterinary sector.

The following areas will expand in the next few years:

- An association between luxury and high-quality medicine.
- Self-diagnosis and self-medication; users will find it very easy to ask for opinions and consultations through online search engines and pharmacies. These platforms will experience intense development.
- Patients will become more demanding, expecting professional, intimate, rapid, and humane treatment.
- Growth of preventive and antiageing medicine. The possibility of DNA sequencing, autogenous vaccines for treating diseases such as cancer, DNA testing for degenerative diseases, the ability to create patient-tailored organs, genetic screening and engineering for "designer babies", and transplant and graft surgery are a few examples of areas that will grow in this sector. All of these fields will bring forth new business opportunities.
- Alternative medicines will expand exponentially, leading to greater collaboration between different sectors and players in the veterinary industry. There will be more centres offering holistic and energy therapies.

Networks and speed

Real-time and interprofessional communication are on the increase. The concept of real-time medicine will be related to the use of multichannel, social media. Facebook, proprietary video or television channels, or real-time series recorded inside a veterinary clinic, à la Big Brother, will earn the loyalty of and attract income from clients around the world.

1. Multidisciplinary medical teams will emerge and place different professionals in touch with each other. The initial forms are WhatsApp and Facebook groups, but whole communities will appear that help further the medical level of their members.

   Research teams will be created wherein the constituents have different profiles and meet to resolve specific problems. This will give rise to collective intellectual experiences that produce greater velocity in technological innovation across all sectors.

2. The future will also bring us telemedicine and the ability to examine and diagnose animals remotely. The development of robotics, for example, will open the possibility of performing surgery from a different city or implanting chips that send data to doctors online. Thus, telemedicine involves real-time, remote monitoring.
3. It will be far simpler to make referrals and obtain second or third opinions because patients will not always have to travel for the initial appointment. This opens an interesting niche in the market for specialists, as they will not only provide physical examinations but also virtual ones in their online clinics.
4. Development of schools and universities that will train and educate professionals online. Virtual university lecture halls will facilitate people's entry into the working world.

Self-diagnosis and self-medication

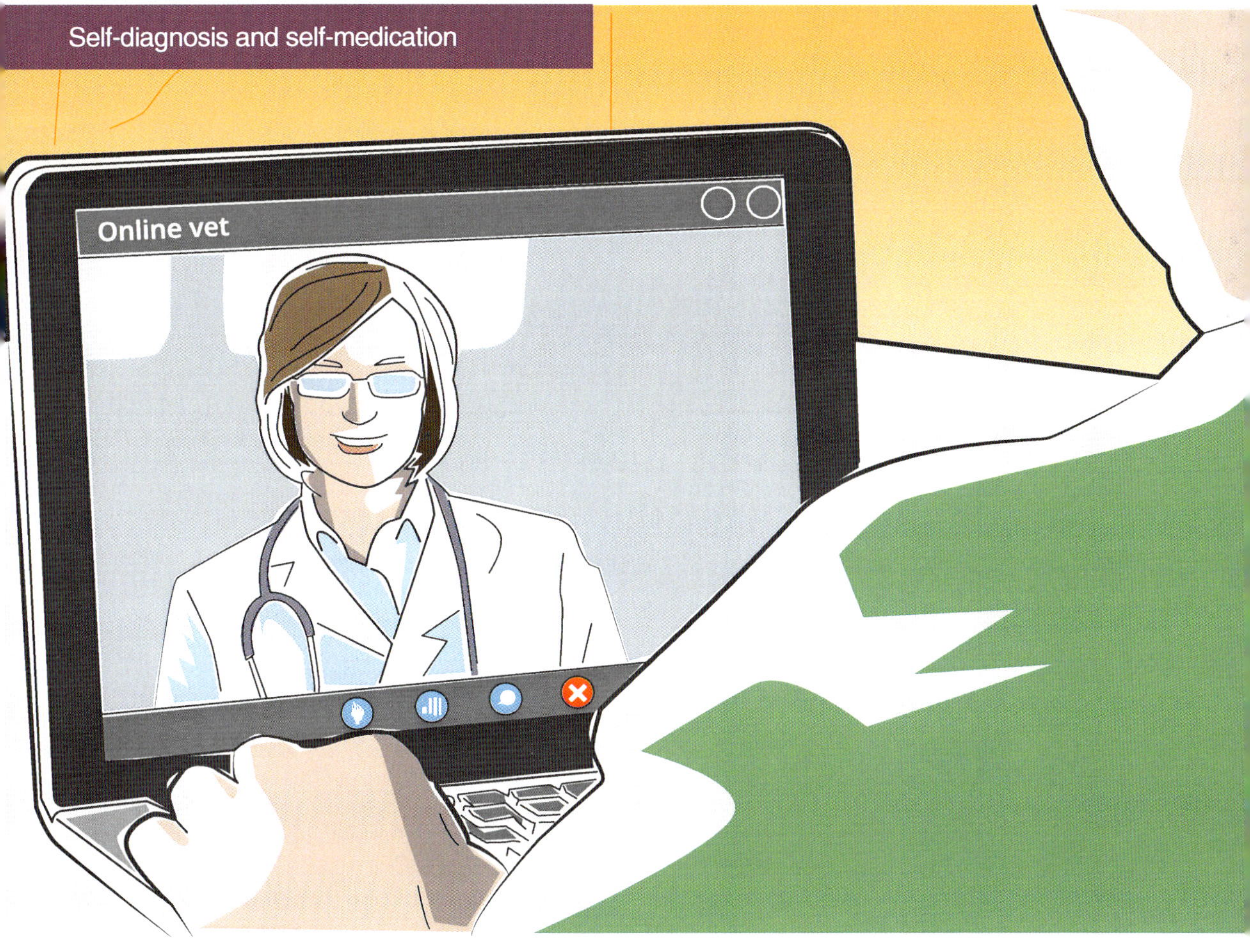

In the veterinary sector

The tendency to invest in healthcare and medicine will increase, as there is a relationship between human and veterinary medicine. Clients will be more demanding and expect higher standards of medical care.

All areas related to accessories, clothes, bags, or beds for pets will also witness significant growth.

Regarding pet food, the trend will be to focus on natural, green, and monoprotein foods, as with human nutrition.

In the coming years, products such as soft drinks or sweets for animals will be developed, alongside new, more complete, and easy-to-administer medications.

Clinics with innovative profiles that recognise these trends early on will gain a competitive edge over more traditional establishments.

**This chapter is based on the excellent book by Pedro Miguel de Sousa Barbosa,* Especulaciones y tendencias (Speculations and Trends), *and the book published by* The Economist, Megachange: The World in 2050.

5 How do your clients perceive you?

Positioning, personal branding, and brands that charm

The image you portray to the consumer depends entirely on you. Generally, there is a certain degree of victimhood in the veterinary world. It is always someone else's fault when things go wrong, or if we find it hard to charge for our labour. Hence the importance of working on your image, so the consumer has a clear idea of your positioning and to establish your personal brand and eventually win over the client.

Positioning

Positioning is knowing your place in the market. Are you the best and most expensive in the city, the cheapest, are you a specialist? Do you know your branding?

Your positioning must be consistent: if you are expensive, you must be really good and provide a high-quality service that matches your rates; if you are cheap, consultations must be brief and efficient, and the agenda must always be full to cover expenses.

Know who you are

Before getting down to business, you have to analyse the field of play (competition and location of the premises), select the desired target market, and assess your strengths and weaknesses to find the ideal position for the veterinary centre.

Learn about your environment

Knowledge is power, that is why information about what the competition offers and the type of clients who will enter your clinic is vitally important. There are two means of ascertaining this information: hire a market research company who will send a mystery shopper to investigate nearby clinics, or do it yourself. A professional will obtain more reliable results, but you could recruit a friend to ask people walking their dogs in parks about which clinics they use and why. The same friend could also visit each of the clinics in your area to request information about the services they provide and their corresponding rates. The results of a survey by one of your friends will probably be biased, yet they will still give you an idea of your market.

Select a path

Do you know your target clients? You cannot please everyone and should not portray a false image of your business. Therefore, depending on your personality, how you work, and your team, you must target the section of the market to which you are most closely aligned. This will provide you with a greater chance of success.

According to neuromarketing studies, the primitive brain rapidly notices when the message is incoherent. If you position yourself as an expert, serious, and rigorous veterinary surgeon via your messages on social media, but in person you actually give off the image of a friendly, customer service-oriented professional, some of the new clients may return but those who expected a more serious, understated treatment may not.

This does not mean you cannot combine solemnity with good service, in fact it is recommendable, but it is true that everyone likes to do business with people who are similar to themselves and we need to see eye to eye before we can reach an agreement. If a client likes serenity, putting an arm around their shoulder, cheerful background music, a brightly lit clinic, or very colourful uniforms may make them feel uncomfortable; and vice versa, more dynamic individuals prefer to enter a clinic that operates flexibly and with a friendly, family atmosphere.

Therefore, you must know what type of client forms your target audience. Messages are better assimilated when they are adapted to the client, you should picture their age, sex, education, family, hobbies, etc. Using a photograph of someone who represents your ideal client is very helpful. It is true that not all clients will conform to this cliché. In fact, most clinics normally have three or four client profiles and therefore you need to create three or four different messages to reach all of them.

SWOT analysis

This tool is used to take the pulse and establish the starting point for your clinic, it helps identify and achieve your goals. Specifically, a SWOT analysis identifies the strengths, weaknesses, opportunities, and threats associated with your veterinary practice.

> A SWOT analysis consists of determining who you are and, consequently, where to position the clinic.

You should always follow the same order: start by analysing the clinic's strengths, then examine the weaknesses. It is always better to exploit what you do well rather than implement new skills, although they are always welcome. After studying the positive and less positive aspects of your clinic you need to look at the threats. With all this information you can identify which opportunities are available.

It is a good idea for each team member to complete the analysis individually before pooling the data and discussing everyone's opinions together. This should be used to create the clinic's overall SWOT analysis.

Mission, vision, and values

This is a method for the brave because it defines your values (or qualities), mission (what you focus on), and vision (your dreams), and it makes a good starting point. It is known as "company culture", since it must endure even though employees come and go.

We recommend starting with the values and mission. Once you have defined these, think about the bigger picture and create the vision: what you want to be.

You can draft these guidelines in a conventional manner and list them separately, or be more creative and form a declaration of principles stating all the information together, or even use an inspirational poem or piece of text that symbolises your ideology to present to your clients. You should make a personal choice about how to do it.

Personal branding

Advertising's worst enemy is indifference. If someone hates you, at least they have you in mind; if they adore you, you have reached the zenith. Indifference implies an inability to influence a potential consumer; no matter how much you try, a disinterested brain will not notice you.

Companies and their brands try to activate the areas in consumers' brains that are connected to pleasure and reward by using different stimuli and effects. Repeating these stimuli helps position their brands as favourites.

Capturing human attention in a multi-impact environment requires significant effort. Impacts achieved through emotions and feelings create the most memories, so large brands work in this direction to try to influence consumers; however, at the same time, overstimulation of the brain leads to indifference. The influences we currently receive from different channels (television, internet, emails, newsletters, WhatsApp, social media) cause the brain to disconnect from what the advertising is trying to accomplish: grabbing our attention through different strategies, such as the surprise effect.

Favourite brands seem to be associated with the right parietal cortex, but there is no specific storage area as up to 75 different locations are involved. Each brand image is encoded along with a network of associations specific to each person; some people are more susceptible to colours, while in others it could be shapes or a memory. In summary, two people loyal to the same brand will not store it in the same area of their cortex because a brand is more than just a logo, top product, or advertising jingle. In fact, nowadays, a brand is a sentiment, what people think about it, what it makes us feel.

Sensory marketing, music, odours, colours, all transform and translate into an experience – your brand.

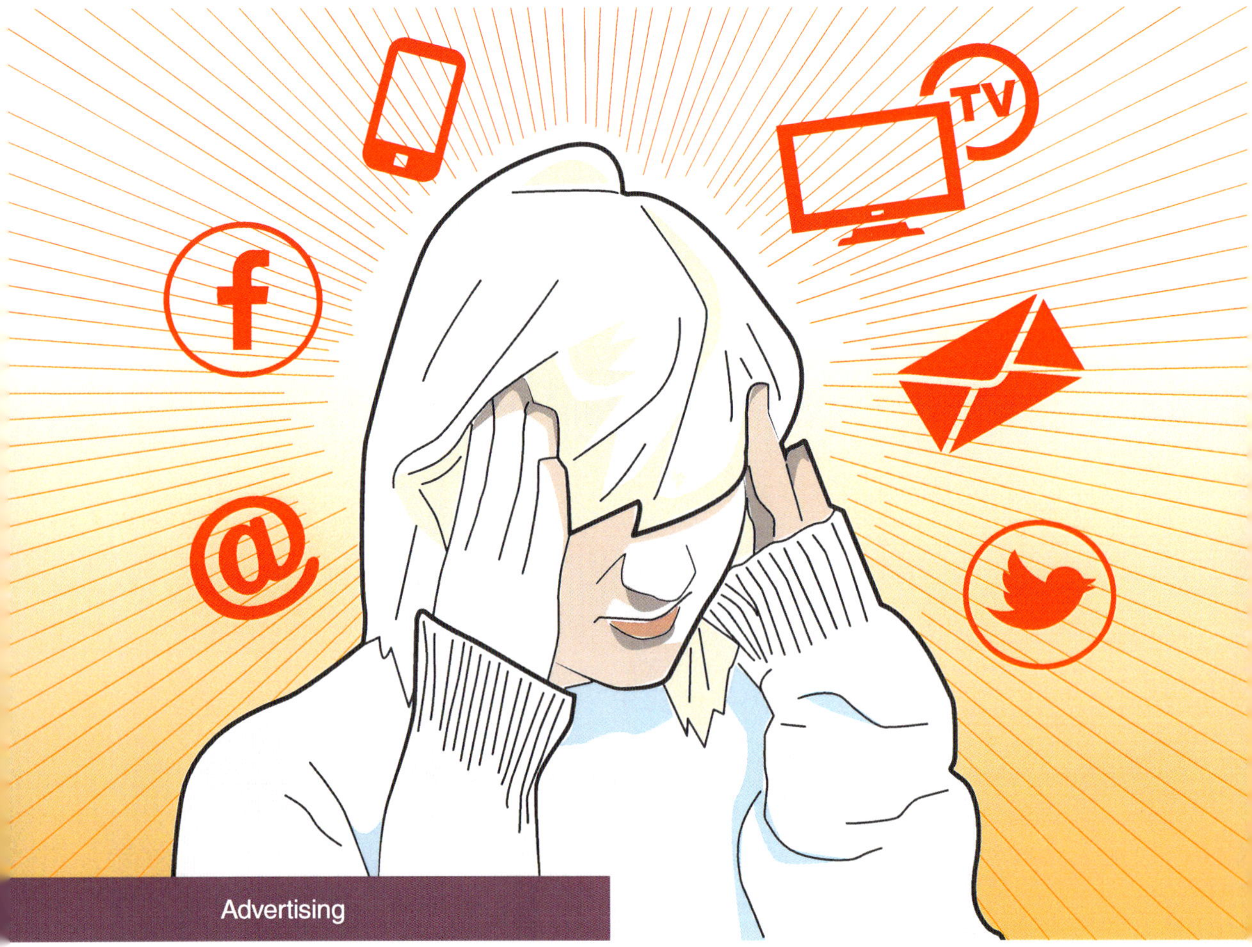

Sell your experience

Your client assumes, although it may be a false premise, that you are going to cure their pet. Since you are a veterinary surgeon, they expect you to resolve their pet's problem. We all know that it is not always possible, but the average client is unaware of this fact.

What the owner can assess is the experience, how you minimise the physical pain of their four-legged friend on one hand and their own emotional pain on the other. Your aim as a veterinary clinician is to ensure that, no matter what happens during the consultation and despite the economic cost of your services, the client leaves the clinic happier (or comforted if they receive bad news) than when they entered in search of help.

Clients find it hard to differentiate between most products and services, but a fitting and memorable experience will guarantee they attribute a greater value to the product or service and are willing to pay more for it. If you really manage to impress your client, they will also tell their friends.

Build a relationship with the client

A relationship involves two parties, but it is the client who decides to initiate it. In fact, as a vet, you unveil yourself to potential clients by creating an internet presence, then they take the first step after deciding to use your services. From that point on, both parties are interested in building a mutually beneficial relationship. It is not as simple as it was in the past, when a lethargy towards changing clinics impeded client defections despite being unsatisfied with the service they received. Now everything is more volatile, and it is hard to earn customer loyalty because of the wide range of veterinary products and services available.

Company website

It used to be said that the centre of all your marketing lies in the clinic's website. However, this has now changed and, although a website is irreplaceable, day-to-day business is propelled by current and emerging social media channels. Ideally, your website should feature information of interest which incorporates social media as a point of origin or destination for potential clients. Neat presentation and some engaging content are essential elements when designing your site. Expressions such as, "the best in", "impeccable treatment", or "9 out of 10 clients gave us the maximum score", are not recommended. The client's experience must lead them to this conclusion, not the clinic itself.

Browsing through the website must be simple and intuitive: if browsers can readily find the telephone number, identify your services, or obtain directions to the centre, it will make it a lot easier for them to visit your clinic.

It is better if the home page contains very little text, and this should be accompanied by coherent images of the services performed at the clinic, rather than an endless presentation that nobody reads.

Customer service

Personalise. Make them feel special

The most important word in the dictionary for anyone is their own name. In our primitive brain, we like to feel special every time we consume. This is even more applicable in relation to our pets. Therefore, it is vital that you address your client by their name and mention their pet's name as many times as possible whenever you talk about them. The owner will feel that both themselves and their pet are very important to you.

Do not delay. Do not make the client wait

Replies such as, "in less than 24 hours" or "I'll get in touch with you as soon as possible", are worth very little. The consumer wants immediate answers; if you do not provide them, they will turn to someone else since they only have to open a search engine on their smartphone. Whether preparing an estimate, arranging an appointment, or responding to a negative or positive comment in a forum, you must act quickly.

The client chooses how they communicate with the clinic, your obligation is to make yourself available to resolve their problems. A few years ago, it was hard to imagine that we could schedule appointments with tools such as WhatsApp or Facebook, yet they are now just another means of communicating and doing business. You must pay attention to the new instruments offered by technology and make them available to your clients.

Simplify. Be accessible and natural

Nobody likes to complete a long form to gain access to you. Try to eliminate barriers to ensure smooth communication with your clients. Gathering information during conversations and recording it in your database will allow you to profile your clients without being bothersome.

Social media reputation

As with relationships, reputations are built or earned, so you must take every opportunity to improve yours. Invite your clients to rate your service on Facebook and Google as soon as you finish the appointment, they will probably oblige. This is simple, free, and very effective, but can reputation be measured?

Measure the client's experience

Philip Kotler said, "The best advertising is done by satisfied customers." How can we measure this satisfaction?

We could write a book just about questionnaires, but with a focus on neuromarketing what we want to learn about are feelings rather than data, tendencies instead of percentages, and something simple is more useful and practical than a 100-item questionnaire.

Hence, here we shall employ something called the Net Promoter Score, or NPS. The NPS is a straightforward means of rating your service as it puts just one question to the client, "On a scale of 0 to 10, what is the likelihood you would recommend XXX veterinary clinic to your friends and acquaintances?"

Those who give you a rating of 9 or 10 are your satisfied clients, to the point where they will happily return to your clinic and actively recommend you to others. These clients are known as promoters of your service, they enhance your reputation. A score of 7 or 8 means they liked the service but are not great fans of your clinic and could succumb to the charms of your competition, these are known as passive clients. Finally, a score of 0 to 6 indicates a dissatisfied client who will probably speak negatively on social media about their experience of your services and will not return to your centre. This last group are labelled as detractors.

The NPS score is calculated by subtracting the percentage of detractors from the percentage of promoters. For example, if 45 % are promoters, 20 % are passive, and 35 % are detractors, the NPS would be 45 – 35 = 10 %.

Anything above 50 % is an excellent score (e.g. Apple is close to 80 %), but the most important thing is to achieve a positive rating, that is, any value above 0 %.

However, we do not have advertising professionals at our disposal. Can vets create a brand? Can we talk in terms of neurobrands? What are the key issues?

How do you create a neurobrand?

Let us establish five stages for building a brand from a neuromarketing point of view:

- Stage 1. Grab the client's attention.
- Stage 2. Build a powerful world view that impacts on the consumer's brain and generates brand loyalty.
- Stage 3. Indulge the senses.
- Stage 4. Work on the client's experience.
- Stage 5. Create client stories, connections, and loyalty. Brands that charm.

Stage 1. Grab the client's attention

The image you portray to the consumer depends entirely on you. As mentioned earlier, you must know who you are and whose attention you seek. The choice of practice type and location are key factors.

If the centre is located in a rural setting, then opening a high-tech clinic may not be the best option. If you decide to open a centre in an upper-class neighbourhood, the installations should be compatible with this environment.

Facilities, packaging, and means of communication must be aligned to the same plan.

In the past, our circumstances were stable and things changed very slowly. Businesses lasted for decades and were passed down to the next generation who could continue to make a risk-free living from them. This has changed, as we currently live in the context of liquid modernity, a term coined by Zygmunt Bauman. It refers to the fact that liquids constantly change shape when placed under tension and adapt to the container holding them. Bauman applies this analogy to the business world and suggests we must build changeable structures in this setting of liquid modernity, that is, companies that adjust to their environment rapidly. The appearance of new ways of doing business and the downfall of old working methods will bring about the closure of many traditional companies if they are unable to accommodate the consumer's ever-changing demands.

Stage 2. Build a powerful world view that impacts on the consumer's brain and generates brand loyalty.

The human mind thinks by creating stories. When a client brings their sick animal to your clinic, their mental narrative pictures the animal returning home and asking for food or running in the park.

Emotional bonds are very important in the setting of a small animal veterinary clinic because in many respects owners assume a parent–child relationship with their pets. Therefore, your reactions and the way you treat the owners are measured in a stressful environment where cognitive biases will play a significant role, as we shall see in Chapter 11.

To start building a world view and creating a narrative, you should begin with the positioning you selected based on the SWOT analysis and company culture (mission, vision, and values).

Your company culture must be reflected in your use of target audience-oriented language, for example if you own a referral centre for other clinics your public will be veterinary professionals. A family clinic, however, can use less formal communication to promote their campaigns or report interesting stories that happen in the neighbourhood.

You should exploit the capacity of social media to create myths and stories. Stories with happy endings (especially when presented as videos) are very powerful and pull on the consumer's heartstrings.

Stage 3. Indulge the senses

Other chapters of this book will deal with this issue in more detail, particularly regarding the waiting room and first impressions. However, when building a brand, the most important point is to develop a multisensory experience. Consumers must like the product's (or service's) colour, presentation, smell, feel, taste, etc. For example, photography enthusiasts are generally fans of either Canon or Nikon, wherein their perception of quality and love for either product depends on factors such as camera weight, the shutter's click, or colour.

Stage 4. Work on the client's experience

The client must feel that what they receive exceeds their expectations. This marks the difference in terms of obtaining customer satisfaction. However, in the 21st century, in a globalised and competitive world, there will always be someone who does the same as you but cheaper. In 1999, Pine and Gilmore said, "Work is theatre and each business a stage." You should aim to create a stage that is so different and attractive it can compete with the sector's heavyweights.

Each business model has a series of advantages and disadvantages. In theory, a small company can adapt and implement changes more readily since, in some ways, its small structure makes it more flexible. It is harder to implement changes in large companies as they comprise many employees and have greater cost structures, so they spend a lot of time processing information gathered from pilot centres before putting innovations into practice across the board. They enjoy the competitive advantage of launching more thoroughly tested products or services which are usually more profitable than those launched by small companies.

Remember: it is not the strongest who survives,
but rather whoever adapts better.

Stage 5. Create client stories, connections, and loyalty

Brands that charm

There is just one more step before attaining success, the one that distinguishes the good from the excellent. The aim is to win your client's heart. You must remember that the public does not buy what you do but rather why you do it. As Blaise Pascal said, "We know the truth, not only by the reason, but also by the heart."

Developing stories at key moments in the consultation ensures the owner feels you are genuinely worried about their animal, so acknowledging their trust and the effort they make for their pet are the most important tools available to you during an appointment.

Once they recognise the role of the clinic, and the established path of the personal brand, the next thing is to make sure the client thinks about your clinic every time they deal with a pet-related issue. Whether you provide a given service or not, your aim is for them to seek your advice before they decide. Admittedly, this is a challenge, but you will learn that it is possible with the following neuromarketing tools and strategies.

Neuromarketing tools and strategies

Lead your team

You must choose between being a boss or a leader. A leader is the first to set the ball rolling, with their example, and triggers a magical chain reaction – imitation.

If the leader gives 100 % to the client,
the staff will be compelled to do the same.

Everything most certainly starts with the selection of the right staff for the clinic, because attitude cannot be trained (they either have it or they do not), but it is also true that if employees with a good attitude observe apathy in their leader, it will eventually rub off on them. Being the boss is more comfortable, but less profitable.

If you look after your team, they will look after your clients

Do you know the names of your employees' parents? Do you know what their hobbies are? Do you eat out together several times a year? Would they tell you about a personal problem?

Your coworkers are, or should be, more than just colleagues. You spend more time with them than with your family and ideally you should enjoy a solid relationship. Not necessarily intimate friendship, but there should be a warm bond. You must do everything possible to ensure they are happy in the clinic and help them achieve their professional objectives (and personal ones if it is within your power). They will fulfil their duties better when they are happy.

Operate in 24-hour mode

If you want to be special, your five senses must be switched on 24 hours a day. You, and each of your employees at the clinic, form your brand, and you must seize every opportunity to politely discuss your work. For example, include your company

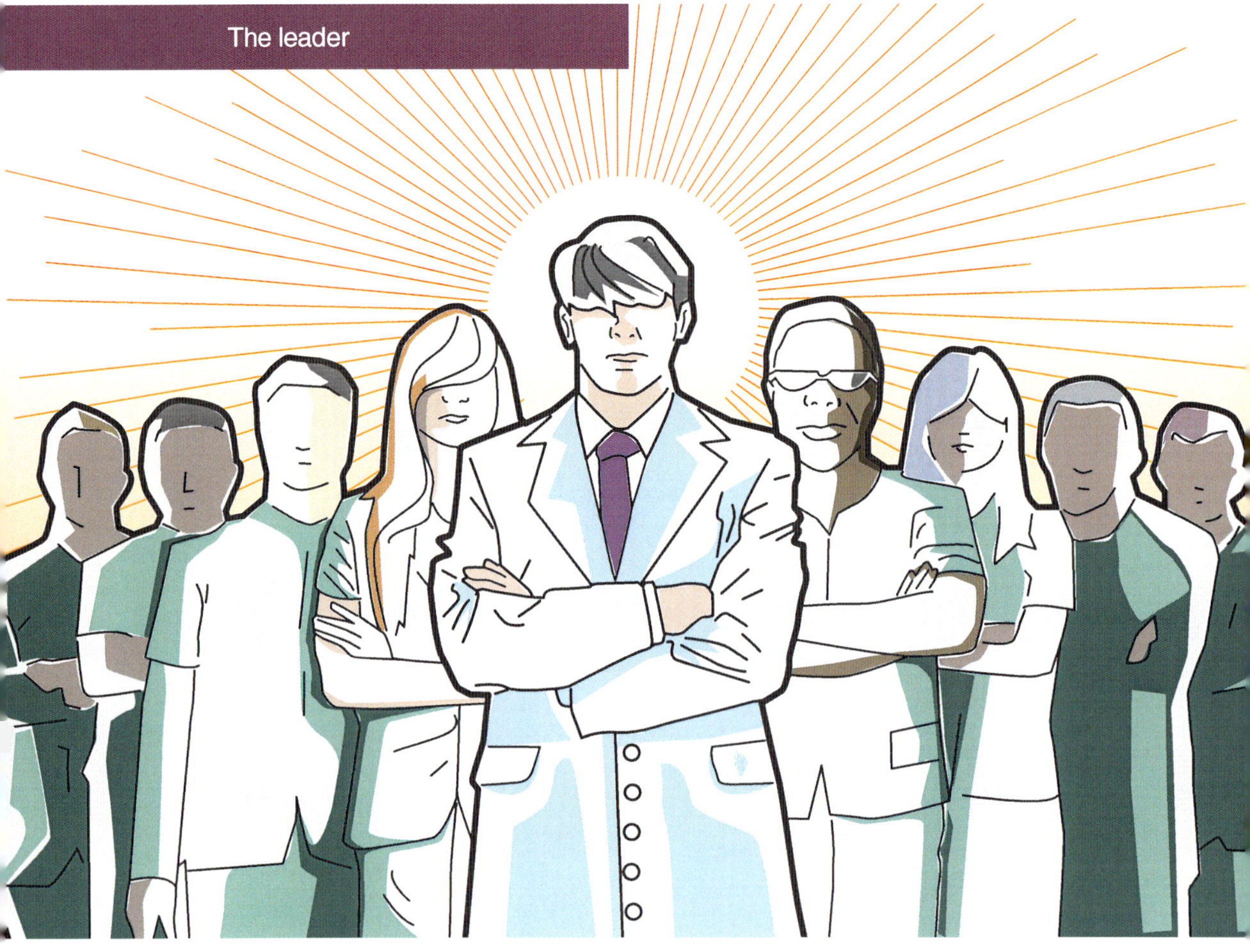

website in the digital signature of all your emails, or remind your clients after each appointment that they can contact you through the emergency telephone number, or if you are called to a parents' meeting for your child's football team, reply that you will be there as soon as you leave your veterinary clinic. Taking advantage of every chance to talk about your clinic will reinforce your brand.

The "wow" effect

"Do what you do so well that they will want to see it again and bring their friends," Walt Disney. Without realising it, Disney was one of the first to use the "wow" effect, which was later popularised by the CEO of Zappos shoes, Tony Hsieh. It entails surprising your customer every time they come into contact with your business, even if they request something unrelated to the services offered by your clinic.

Amongst other characteristics, a service with "wow" factor should:

- Be fun and offbeat.
- Be creative, adventurous, and open-minded.
- Do more with less.
- Build a positive team with a family spirit.
- Pursue growth and learning.
- Be enthusiastic and determined.
- Build open, honest relationships.
- Be humble.
- Adopt and promote change.

This implies that all team members give everything they've got during each contact with a client, so that the client does not leave the centre feeling indifferent. Each team member should grasp every appointment as an opportunity to shine, so the client finds it almost impossible to consider changing clinic.

As a practical exercise, visualise your average consultation and assess each point of contact (touchpoint) between you and the client: the information they find on the internet including your website and previous clients' reviews, the telephone call to make an appointment, their arrival at the centre and parking their car, entry to the clinic and the way the client and patient are received, the consultation itself, the payment process, arranging a new appointment, and departure. In your own view, rate each touchpoint from 1 to 10 and join the dots. The objective is to address the points with the lowest scores and obtain a clear idea of where you can improve to ensure each client experiences the "wow" effect at their next visit.

Surf the wave of change

You can either crash against the wave or try to surf it. One thing is for sure, the waves are unremitting. Change is hardwired into consumer culture and veterinary clinics, just like any other business, must adapt to it. In fact ideally they should promote change.

Steve Jobs said that people did not realise they needed an iPhone until he introduced them. You can imitate successful models, but you will always be one step behind their creators; or you can develop a special model that makes your client fall in love, either because of the service's technical features or the way you present and execute it.

CHARMING IDEAS

- Address the client and their pet by their names. Humans like to hear their name more than any other word.
- Be creative, improvise when faced with unexpected situations.
- Adapt to change and promote innovation. It is better to create than copy.
- If there is a problem, act. The one thing you must avoid is passivity.
- Try to create the "wow" effect during each visit.
- Always consider how you would like to be treated in each situation.

6 Are you willing to change?

*"We are not thinking machines with emotions,
we are emotional machines with thoughts."
Dámaso Alonso.*

There is no easy answer because carrying on as you are is always very comfortable. Therefore, before talking about change, we shall explain automatic pathways, brain plasticity, and the different types of memory.

Automatic pathways

A 20-year-old's brain weighs approximately 1.3 kg. Unlike all other organ's in the human body, the brain shrinks as we get older. Along with the spinal cord, a long tube-like structure that emerges from the brainstem and tapers down the spine, the brain comprises the physical centre of human behaviour. Although it corresponds to less than 2 % of our body weight, it consumes around 30 % of available energy. Hence it is very costly to maintain and therefore automatic pathways are established to minimise energy consumption.

Neurons, the basic unit of the nervous system, are connected by synapses. The repetition and fortification of neural routes helps entrench pathways and maps. As we said before, this process requires a lot of energy expenditure, so automatisms are created.

An automatic mechanism saves energy; however, the brain must develop new routes or synapses to learn something new and this costs a lot of energy.

So, learning is an energy-sapping exercise that costs more as we get older. That is why it is much easier to learn a language in early childhood rather than above the age of 40, because adults need to make an extra effort.

Brain plasticity

Brain plasticity, also known as neuroplasticity, is the ability to learn and create new pathways, as well as the ability to change opinion, something which also deteriorates with age.

Everyone perceives the world differently and acts according to their life experiences. This is what forms the distinction between identical twins who share the same genetics but have been exposed to different experiences.

We receive a constant stream of information, even when asleep, which translates into a series of actions that influence our lives, modify our surroundings, and form our brains.

Just like plastic, the brain adapts to almost anything, it shapes our experiences and uses them to interpret situations we may encounter in the future.

Types of memory

Memory can be classified into two types: short- and long-term memory. Short-term memory, or working memory, is the immediate retention of information for 5 to 6 hours before it is forgotten; long-term memory is lifetime retention of information. Self-concept, and who we are, is associated with long-term memory. Memory has a special relationship with sentiment, to such an extent that we remember emotional material better than cognitive. That is why brands always allude to feelings and we talk about experiential marketing.

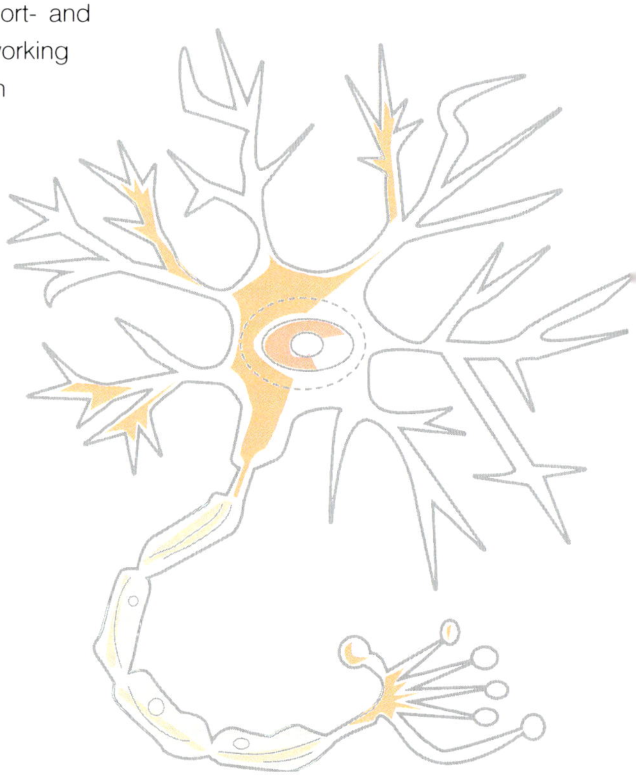

We employ a series of automatic pathways, or routines, during work and everyday life to simplify our daily chores. These routines mean there is no need to fully concentrate on what we are doing. Both the cerebral cortex and cerebellum are involved in these automatisms. How many times have you driven home almost without even realising it because you were thinking about other things? The cerebellum takes care of the automatisms, although the brain is monitoring for any unexpected events.

When the brain is faced with any suggestion of change, it immediately and automatically reacts by refusing to accept it. The brain does not want to undergo changes and resists them. So, you must learn to overcome this "inner self" when attempting to do things differently.

Consequently, it is quite normal for both you and your staff to experience internal resistance when you start to apply neuromarketing in your clinic. These factors must be considered because sales techniques should be implemented collectively and therefore all personnel must be involved before establishing a new technique.

Business models

In the past, vets would open a centre and gradually incorporate new team members and knowledge, while also improving their facilities. Even so, a veterinary clinic was a stable business in which clients had to wait for an appointment and practitioners did not need to know a lot about marketing and sales. Practices were often exclusive to the area and new clients entered under their own steam, they had no other option. The clinics fulfilled a need. Furthermore, the stability of these businesses meant they could be passed down from parents to children and employees completed many years of service; staff turnover was very low. This is the classic 20th century model, that of a very traditional, stable business. It is a market-oriented model.

However, trends have changed in the 21st century with the emergence of highly changeable environments and the liquid economy. We refer to technological changes and the need to adapt to the times. The number of veterinary practices has increased exponentially, so the client can easily take their business to a new clinic if they are unsatisfied.

We are witnessing the advent of new ways of doing business, corporations and large centres that set up chains of clinics, franchises, hospitals, referral centres, university centres, and the ever-present local veterinary clinic. Clients find it very hard to decide which centre best suits their needs, hence they rely on 21st century word of mouth, in other words, social media and opinion forums.

Against this backdrop, the need arises to position the client in the centre of the service, as this will differentiate one clinic from another. Excellence in customer care, communication, and how you present your products and services and earn client loyalty, force you to pursue constant evolution within your company. This is a client-oriented model.

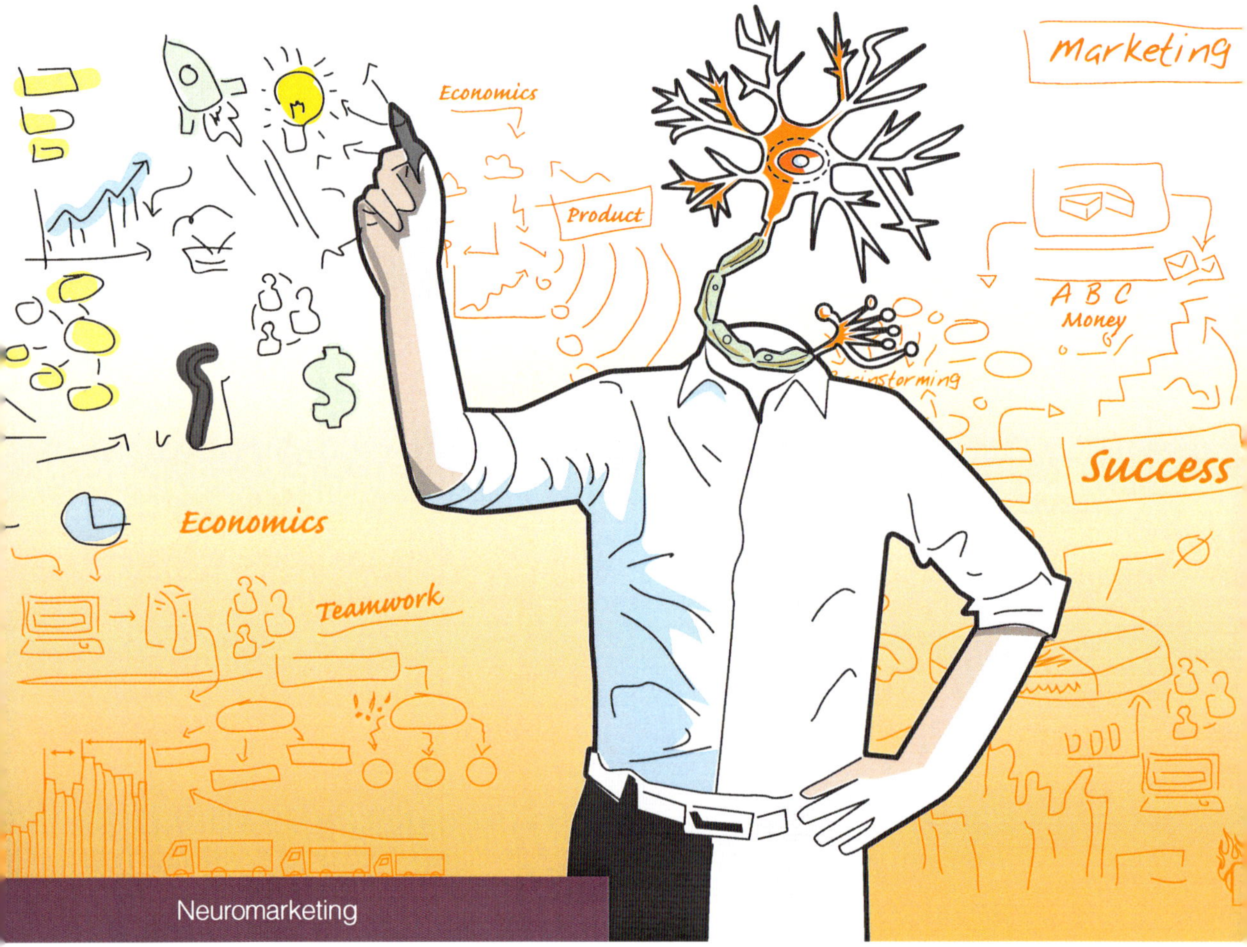

Neuromarketing

The first business model was a very traditional concept, which never placed the customer at the centre of the sales process. It was based on a paternalistic image of the veterinary surgeon, where the specialist made all the decisions without seeking the owner's opinion or consensus. The vets were always the ones who thought about the treatment, facilities, prices, and competition. In the 21st century, since the client and pet have been placed at the centre of the business, neuromarketing has proven a very practical and easy-to-implement tool, while it demonstrates that purchasing mechanisms are more emotional than rational. The firm bond clients have with their animals means these easily applied techniques have a strong impact for the vet.

Neuromarketing

Neuromarketing is the study of purchasing and brand loyalty mechanisms, thus providing a new frame of reference. Applied to the veterinary sector, it shifts our vision of the company and that of the professional because it focuses the entire business around the way the vet communicates with their clients in order to earn their approval and treat the patients.

Currently, to develop a successful veterinary clinic, you must concentrate on fulfilling several aspects:

- Client-oriented company. We shall discuss how to design the waiting room or consultation room from a neuromarketing perspective.
- Client-oriented consultation. You must establish a trust-based relationship with the client before you can perform good veterinary practice. If you do not earn their trust, you cannot realise your job properly. That is where neuromarketing comes in.
- How to offer your services.
- Using neuromarketing to connect with clients through social media.
- Client-oriented telephone skills. Use the telephone as a loyalty-building tool.
- Focus on your employees. They are known as your internal clients.

The market changes rapidly, so it is hardly surprising that new business models are constantly emerging, some of which are truly disruptive. Most companies we are familiar with today did not exist less than a century ago. The same is true looking back over the last 25 years, for example, the music, tourism, and telecommunication industries have undergone radical changes. In the veterinary sector, the rural vet has all but disappeared and been replaced by small animal veterinary clinics.

The technological revolution will trigger the arrival of novel models for veterinary practices, to such an extent that the next 25 years will see the creation of a multitude of entirely new job positions.

The advent of telemedicine and remote diagnosis is erasing physical barriers, but veterinary clinics have always been conceived as local businesses and therefore you will need to broaden your strategies to attract clients to your practice.

A common characteristic of successful companies is they are driven by what people want and use technologies to accelerate procedures. The world is entering a new era.

Neuroscience is allowing companies to get inside the consumer's mind, they are learning the art of mental seduction. Some of the mechanisms are executed instinctively, which is why they say a salesperson is born and not made.

One of the main advantages inherent to the veterinary sector is the strong emotional tie between owners and their pets. This connection is created by building bonds of trust and improving communication skills. It will allow you to work to the best of your abilities.

What do salespeople from different sectors have in common?

Above all, they create trust because they believe in what they are doing and know how to transmit this belief, thus generating loyalty and the likelihood of being recommended to potential new clients.

We are witnessing a new era in terms of business models, and veterinary clinics, as one of the agents in the pet industry, must know how to adapt to this modern period.

Everything sold, bought, and communicated will be recorded in powerful CRM software; we are in the age of digitalisation where video-conferences and augmented reality can produce a large shift in the sector and everyday working methods.

Have you considered how flexible you are in the face of change? How much "chameleon potential" does your business have? Are you prepared to understand your new, more emotional client? Are you willing to change and learn to apply neurosales techniques to offer your services?

If you are willing, you will find the keys to achieving these goals in the following chapters.

7 Sell – what a wretched word!

We are all salespeople and, like it or not, we sell on a daily basis. We sell and offer our best version to our friends, or when going on a date as you dress up to look sexy or feel attractive. We all sell ourselves. We sell ourselves because we want others to notice us and speak positively about us.

We may be good or bad at selling ourselves, but we can always control the type of image we wish to portray or impression we want to cause. Therefore, it is better to control certain situations rather than leave them to chance.

Some people are born with an innate ability to sell; they are communicative, cheerful, good listeners, and know how to interpret what the speaker needs.

However, the sales process can be learnt and developed further. When we learn a technique that gives positive results, the mind automatises the method, so it will be easier to repeat the next time.

We also sell our services in the clinic: through our telephone skills, with the correct greeting or a smile; we now know that these factors have an impact on purchasing decisions. A good presence sells, as does our team. Equally, a bad response from one of our assistants could cause us to lose a loyal client.

EXAMPLE

The first thing a new parent does is take their tightly wrapped baby to the doctor, so they can hear that everything is okay; some even do this every week. The first time you take your child to the paediatrician, you do not imagine they will say, "What an extraordinarily ugly child, he looks like a lizard." In your mind you would form the idea, "If this doctor doesn't like children, why did they become a paediatrician?" and you would never return to the centre.

In the given example, medical criteria were not considered, it would be an emotional decision because that is how parents would understand the situation before them. If a parent takes their offspring, which they see as the most perfect being on earth, to a doctor who treats them in a manner they consider inappropriate, it would lead them to conclude this paediatrician is the worst person in the world. Having said that, we each assess the attention received according to our own parameters. A doctor would rate it in line with their experience as a healthcare professional, but most clients are neither doctors nor vets, so they will primarily assess you in function of well-known and emotional factors: first impression, greeting, cleanliness, friendliness, and what is more they will discuss these points with others.

You need to decide whether you want to control how you sell. This will define how successful the sale turns out to be.

Which criteria do people base their decisions on? What are the elements of communication?

You should select your own phrases or criteria depending on your personality, experiences, and nature. There are no magic expressions, rather you must learn to observe and read your clients.

The foundations of traditional sales techniques talk about specific phrases that help us sell more than any other, but in practice, we each have to develop our own language.

It is not a question of either a rational or totally emotional sale, you must be able to identify the current behavioural pattern of the person standing before you and know how to adjust instantly. It is therefore important to learn how to consciously read people's body language.

EXAMPLE

If you were going to buy a pair of shoes, the salesperson would ask what you wanted them for, whether they were for everyday use or a special occasion. This is a good way of establishing the first point of communication. Telling a brief story produces an image in the consumer's mind which makes them think about their purchase, therein lies the success of storytelling: we think through stories and images. In the present example, the consumer will imagine wearing the chosen shoes to the special occasion.

If the staff at your veterinary centre can elicit emotions as soon as your clients enter, they will have already established a significant amount of trust. The personal stories you frequently hear in the clinic are those which create bonds. Asking about the story of a dog the client has taken in from a shelter or the particular situation of a relative who has lost a pet are examples of how to connect with the client's mind.

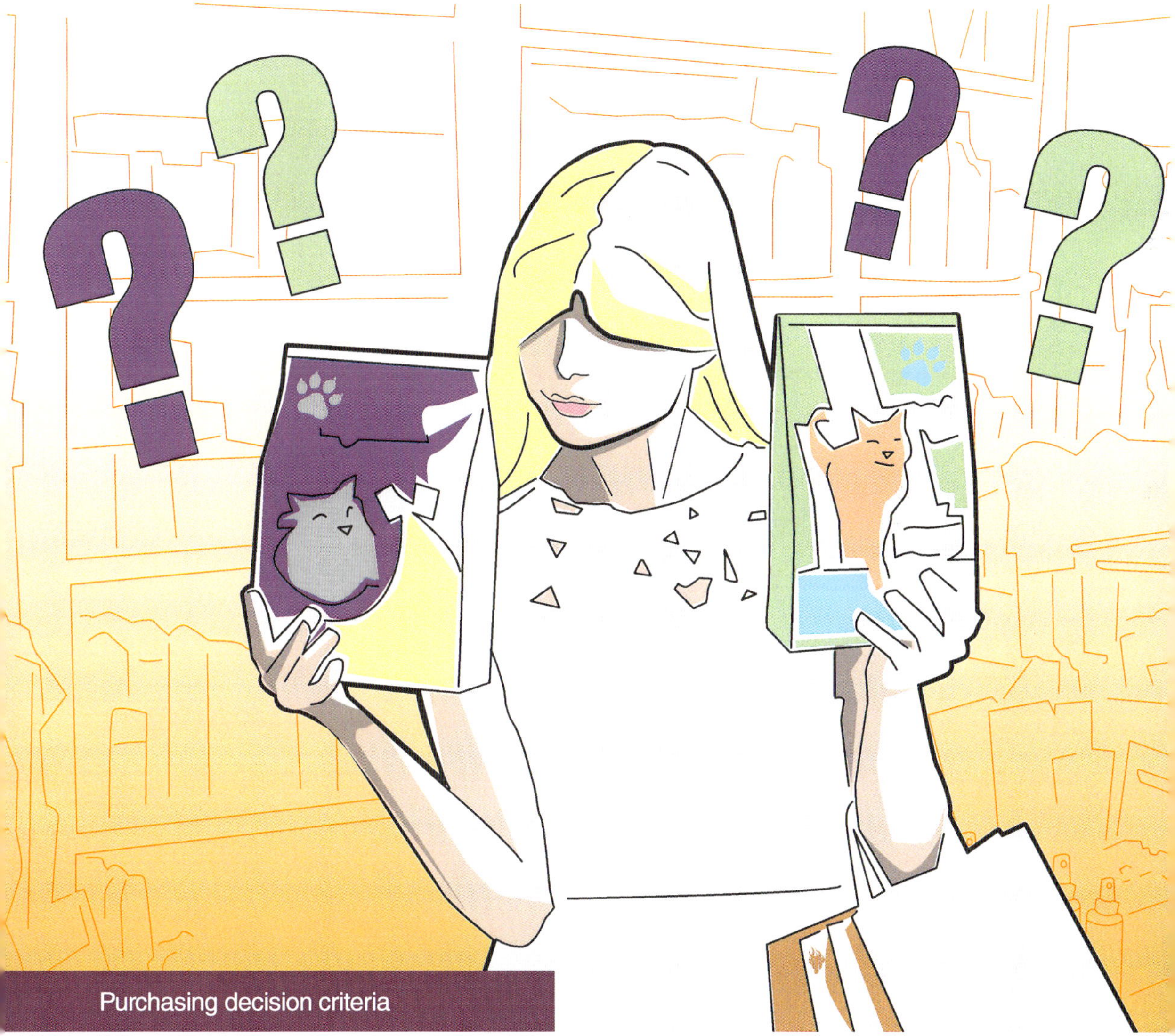

Purchasing decision criteria

In our case, as vets we must learn to use our work to generate value in the eyes of others. This means that details such as remembering the patient's and client's names are essential when it comes to building relationships.

Never forget what lies behind each patient; a family whose circumstances you must discover through a trust-based relationship in order to give the animal the best possible veterinary care.

The emotion the veterinary surgeon stimulates when talking is a key selling point, even if the feelings are created rationally. To be honest, we do not know why people buy things, as 85 % of the purchasing process is carried out subconsciously, but we do know that everyone likes to appear intelligent and therefore we justify what we do.

"Sell it to the mind, not the people."
Jürgen Klarić

You must sell without selling because the secret of sales is listening. Your aim during a consultation is to listen and determine what the client perceives as the problem.

EXAMPLE

Occasionally the owner visits the clinic because their dog has conjunctivitis, but they also have clear signs of truncal alopecia and the vet has just completed a training course in dermatology, so it represents a very interesting opportunity to apply their newly acquired knowledge. When the owner explains the dog has been losing hair for 8 months, the vet starts to talk excitedly about the dog's skin, but that is not the problem in the owner's eyes, it is not their reason for visiting the clinic. The client had a dog that went blind, so what they are really worried about is the same thing happening to Bobby. Their fear is related to Bobby's eyesight, not his skin. The vet must address and resolve the eye condition, then make another appointment to follow-up on the eye in which they can mention the dog's skin, but after having gained the client's trust by providing the peace of mind that Bobby is not going to go blind. If, on the other hand, the vet focuses on the skin problem and recommends some tests to obtain a thyroid profile, the owner will feel uncomfortable and unreceptive to these tests because they took Bobby to the clinic to treat his eye problem.

The mind finds it easier to rule things out than to decide, and you should be acutely aware of this point when explaining diagnostic protocols to the owner. In the previous example, by pushing the client towards the skin problem rather than resolving the conjunctivitis, the vet would have created psychological discomfort resulting in the client declining to progress with a future diagnosis of the skin condition.

To summarise this chapter, the following is a checklist of the points a neurosalesperson must bear in mind:

POINTS TO CONSIDER FOR THE NEUROSALESPERSON

1. Ensure you listen actively. Observe and make a quick assessment of the client's body language.
2. Use your whole body to communicate: face, hands, gestures, and body position.
3. Use your voice and acoustic modelling (paralanguage).
4. Analyse and adapt to the type of consumer. Use mirror neurons.
5. Listen to and focus on what the client has to say. Resolve the problem which has brought the client to your clinic.
6. Remember that people make emotional purchases and the "fear factor" is very important for clients.
7. Reduce the client's level of stress because it can impede the decision-making brain.
8. Explain information using the clearest language possible for the listener and minimise the use of veterinary terms. If veterinary terminology is required, "translate" the terms so they can understand them.
9. Help the owner decide by defending the patient.
10. Use stories and accounts to explain the expected benefits of any tests you recommend. Narrate a story. Carry out this entire process consciously, applying your knowledge and, where possible, following a protocol.

8 Attracting clients. Reputation, coherence, and symbolic value

The access points to the veterinary clinic

In most clinics, 80 % of clients enter because of the centre's proximity, apart from the case of referral practices which have a wider area of influence.

Veterinary clinics have a range of access points:

- **Physical entrance**. The pet owner walks directly into your clinic. The first thing they see is the façade, followed by the reception.
- **Telephone**. The potential user contacts you by telephone, requesting information, a price estimate, or an appointment.
- **Offline reputation**. The owner of a new pet asks their acquaintances for recommendations.
- **Social media**. This is an increasingly important entry channel because the user can independently investigate your website, company, reputation, and the opinions of other clients. You must learn how to manage your social media channels and online reputation as you do your offline life.

You must work on three aspects to attract new clients:

1. Reputation.
2. Coherence.
3. Symbolic value of your product.

How does neuromarketing influence these access points?

1. Reputation

The opinion, view, or concept that people have about something: a person, a thing, or, in our case, a company.

A good reputation is one of your differential advantages over your competition, where the client values both tangible and intangible factors.

Neuromarketing strives to ensure the client develops a positive emotional association with you and recommends your clinic, whether directly or via social media.

This emotional connection is achieved through a multichannel and multisensory process. The association will depend on the client's expectations, which must be exceeded to produce a positive long-term memory. The deeper the sentiment, the deeper the memory. However, you must remember the impact could be negative and by the same token it will create a memory.

If the client receives a level of service in line with their expectations, the recommendation rate will fall because it was nothing special in their eyes.

Whereas, if the service is well below their expectations, they will leave the clinic feeling totally dissatisfied. This is seriously detrimental because, although they might not complain at the clinic, statistically, the client will report this failing in the offline world seven times more than if they had received excellent service. In terms of social media, the impact can be even greater as a single mouse click can share a negative opinion with thousands of people.

SUMMARY

Reputation is earned after hard work, it depends on your efforts over several years. It is obtained throughout the entire service chain and associated with client expectations. Any false move or error can have a negative effect on the client's level of satisfaction, consequently you must be extremely careful at every stage of the chain.
Reputation is also related to coherence, since an incoherent service will create a bad impression.

BASIC CLIENT EXPECTATIONS THAT YOU MUST LOOK AFTER TO MAINTAIN A GOOD REPUTATION

Good access to the clinic and outstanding customer service in reception.

Opening times that suit the client's needs and correlate with the services offered by your clinic.

Reasonable waiting times before the consultation or when paying.

A sense that their problem or need has been addressed, and that you have provided the tools to resolve it.

Close and understandable (avoid too many technical terms) verbal and non-verbal communication with respectful listening. Therefore, answers must be concise, clear, and complete.

Explain what will happen after the consultation, and why you need to schedule another visit.

Always fulfil any promises.

Create a cross-sale that ensures the client has a positive experience.

Improve on the feelings they experienced in another veterinary practice.

The client should feel their pet is being cared for as if it were the vet's own.

Some of the unforeseen reasons why a client's expectations may not be met are:

- Clients may sometimes have unreasonable or disproportionate expectations which you could never meet, this can lead to between 20 % and 30 % of the problems associated with dissatisfaction.
- All team members must be trained how to interpret the client's expectations.
- Marketing campaigns with incomplete or confusing messages can result in disappointment.
- Errors committed by an employee with low motivation or a grievance against the company.

Incomplete or confusing messages in marketing campaigns

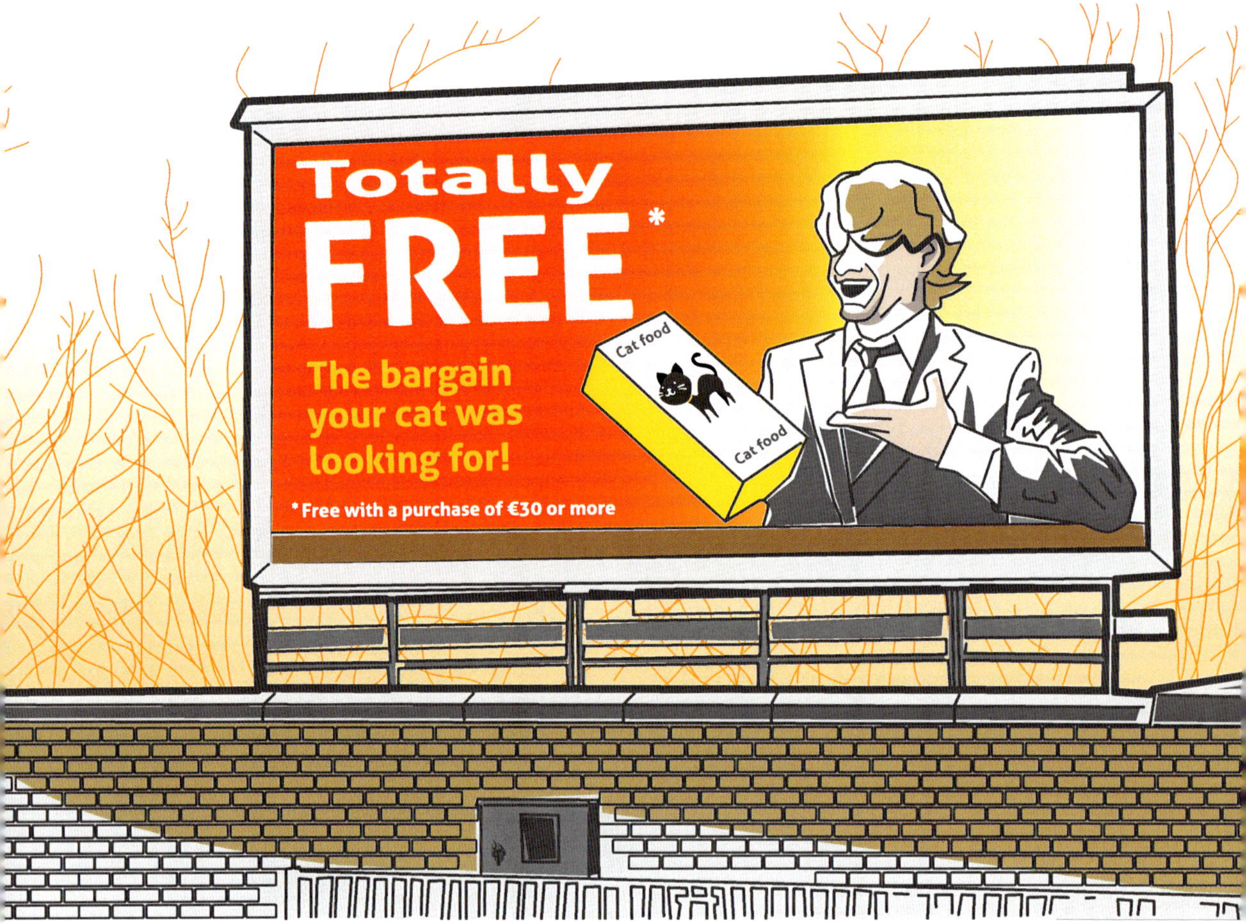
Totally
FREE*
The bargain your cat was looking for!
*Free with a purchase of €30 or more
Cat food
Cat food

To maintain and improve your reputation, you should add this concept to the company's strategic plans, as a poor reputation could increase the number of clients who leave your clinic.

In the case of a recently opened veterinary clinic, it is very important to invest a lot of effort in creating a positive reputation as quickly as possible.

2. Coherence

Coherence is the logical association between two things, parts, or elements of a whole, so that there is no contradiction or conflict between them.

EXAMPLE

Suppose you own a small practice with an old-fashioned waiting room. If you fill your website with photos of high-quality veterinary models and facilities, the client will notice something does not coincide with their expectations as soon as they walk through the door, and their visual impression of the facilities results in discomfort or rejection. This is a clear example of incoherence.

EXAMPLE

The same thing can occur in a large veterinary hospital if the employee who receives a telephone call is curt and does not express concern for the client, or if they are impolite because the reception is very busy. All clients at a veterinary hospital expect an excellent level of personal attention at every stage of the process, otherwise, in their opinion, it would fall short of being a hospital because they did not receive the special attention they anticipated.

When talking about a company's internal coherence, it refers to a converging relationship between the company (image, structure, staff training level, and all other aspects that make up the business) and its ethical principles.

To achieve coherence, the company must define its size, ideal client, niche in the market, and client type.

Your practice must also define its type of veterinary model, since, in both a small clinic or a hospital, the level of veterinary care and customer service must be in harmony with the business structure and will differ in each case. In short, you must be clear about the company's mission, vision, and values.

Company coherence is a multifaceted parameter. For example, if you decide to open a practice in an upper-class neighbourhood, the physical structure, space, design, and shopfront must coincide with the local population's expectations. Yet, when opening a practice in more modest surroundings, you must establish a structure that fits in with the characteristics of the area. Similarly, in a very large veterinary clinic, you may lose proximity with clients, so staff must treat clients with excellent manners. While in a small local clinic, familiarity with patients and their owners is of paramount importance.

At this point the consumer starts to construct a mental picture of price levels. When clients visit a large veterinary hospital, they assume the final bill will be higher than at a smaller clinic. It would be incoherent for a large veterinary hospital to offer inappropriate discount policies, likewise, you would not expect hospital prices at a rural clinic.

In fact, appropriate prices for each business should be defined by the company's fixed costs, not by the competition's prices. The company, its size, and its cost structure are the factors that define a suitable pricing interval. If the calculations produce untenable prices, the company will be incoherent. If, a priori, your rates are tenable, presumably the company will be healthy and highly profitable.

It is surprising that some cafés can charge £5 for a cup of coffee and clients will happily pay, while the same price in other premises would be considered daylight robbery.

Upon entering a restaurant, the client can guess how much the final bill will be based on its location, the waiting list for a reservation, the decoration, and the appearance of the waiting staff. The same applies to veterinary centres.

Coherence emanates a price range that should not give cause for alarm in the consumer's mind. An incoherent company will fail in the marketplace.

Company coherence is not just an external factor emitted to the client, but it is also an internal aspect presented to your staff. This means processes must be well-defined, for example, staff pricing or discount policies, as should issues concerning internal relationships and task allocation. As practices grow, such aspects must be unequivocally defined and clarified, otherwise the company's growth will result in chaos and disorganisation.

A poor working environment is unacceptable when trying to provide high-quality customer service. Clients can detect a good or bad atmosphere as soon as they enter the waiting room, and it is a decisive factor in determining whether they return.

These points are the responsibility of the clinic's manager or owner, who should try to connect these elements, which initially appear to be just sensory, with aspects of good old-fashioned financial management. Neuromarketing is profitable and you must learn to measure it with financial parameters.

3. Symbolic value

Symbolic value depends on sentimentality, the feeling of belonging, and feeling special by forming part of something special, which is the real reason why people buy things.

The symbolic value of an object is its ability to transmit ideas, for example, the Christian cross, the Star of David, or brand trademarks such as the Audi symbol.

Consumers are loyal to products and brands because of what they represent more than what they are. Very strong relational experiences convert a lot of products or companies into idealised brands for consumers. Classic examples are fans of Harley-Davidson motorcycles who get tattoos of their logos, or the passion that Apple induces amongst its devotees and followers. We use the terms devotees and followers because the symbolic value of the product or brand is encompassed in a pseudoreligious symbolism.

- Brands have supporters and advocates (fans of Canon versus those who prefer Nikon), they are disciples because they recommend and try to convince others.
- Brands have symbols (the apple of Apple).
- Brands have leaders and legends (Steve Jobs), and even clothing (Harley-Davidson).
- They have their own temples and shops.
- The decorative elements of a brand's chain of stores share common designs and feel the same, while the client experiences the same odours and colours.

EXAMPLE

What is the symbolic value of a diamond? A diamond sparkles, but so do several types of glass. The symbolic value of a diamond is its power, the certainty it will not lose value, and it indicates the wearer has significant purchasing power; in fact, it is an investment. Ultimately, it represents prestige and security.

Symbolic value

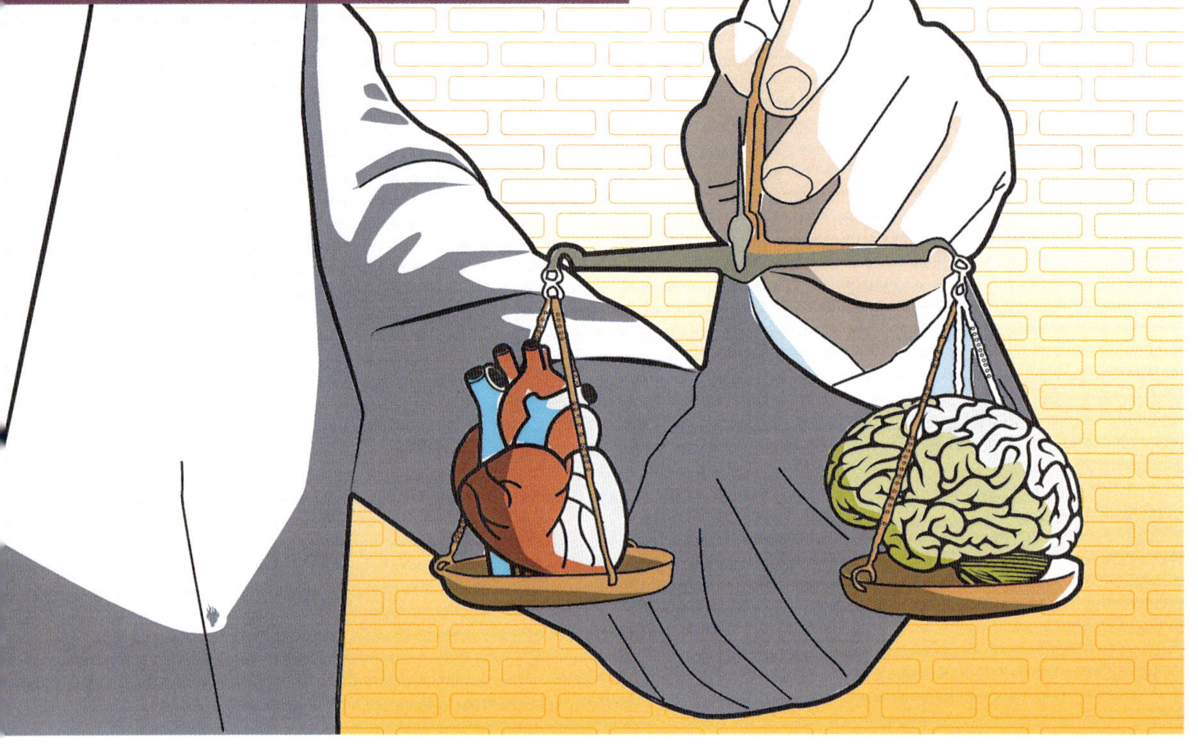

EXAMPLE

What is the symbolic value of a high-end car? The power, size, success, exclusivity, and relative inaccessibility. Humans tend to act like monkeys, we love to be the centre of attention. Luxury brands are very good at manipulating this type of market. It is a sense of a belonging to an elite group, as demonstrated by the fact that there are long waiting lists to purchase handbags.

The symbolic value of veterinary practices

If we analyse what veterinary practices offer, the first idea could be veterinary well-being for the client's pet.

However, after speaking with clients, they report that their relationship with their pets is more like what a parent feels towards a baby. Animals need their owners throughout their entire lives and the pet–owner communication process is one of total dependence. Owners want to be sure they will not lose their furry baby when they visit their vet. How often have you heard clients say the first "person" they greet every morning is their doggy?

That is why you must be able to climb rungs on the ladder of symbolic value, since you are offering more than just veterinary services – you are offering the security of being protected and looking after their furry baby.

If you climb another rung, we discover that people with dogs and other animals are friendlier, more affectionate, happier, and live longer, as revealed by a 2008 study conducted in 4,435 people which concluded that owning a pet cat reduces the risk of suffering a heart attack. Animal lovers are considered to be better, more sensitive, and more emotionally developed people.

As vets we must be aware of the symbolic value that we offer to our public. We can maximise the animal's quality of life and lifespan, which bears an influence on their owner's happiness.

There is a family and a story behind each pet, so are you prepared to accept the challenge of looking after the pet's health and the family's happiness?

To attract clients to your clinic, you must know how to connect with the symbolic value you are offering because new competitors and novel business models with different symbolic values are always emerging. Here are some examples:

- Animal welfare organisations that act as veterinary practices. What is their symbolic value? They connect through the concept of helping animals in need and which have been abused or abandoned.
- Clinics that are highly engaged with respect to caring for the environment. Their symbolic value is based on their relationship with and caring for animals and plants. They should focus on a young public who place great importance on respect for nature. They use renewable energies and are strongly committed to recycling. They could sell, for example, products for carrying pets on bicycles and promote countryside trails. Their symbolic value is environmental care.
- Clinics whose symbolic value focuses on treating animals as family members, establishing a sense of belonging to a club in which people and animals live together.
- Referral centres and large veterinary hospitals. In this case the symbolic value is treatment from specialists and the highest levels of care, which is not within everyone's reach.
- Luxury clinic. The symbolic value is belonging to an elite group.

- Alternative medicine centres for animals, with natural therapies, homeopathic and allopathic medicines, acupuncture, and diet therapy. Their symbolic value is to search for the origins of and use energy-based medicines.
- Mobile veterinary service. Here, the symbolic value is, "you cannot come to me, but I will help you." The client does not have to forsake the happiness of owning a pet because they have limited mobility.
- Therapeutic animals. Their symbolic value is the use of animals as a tool to help improve people's health.
- Large shopping centres. Here the symbolic value is the opportunity to go shopping with your pet. There is a large variety of products to choose from and the symbolic value is the client's dedication to their pet and the opportunity to go shopping together.
- Low-cost practices. Their symbolic value is offering services at a cheaper rate than the competition: "Do not waste your money anywhere else."

TIP

You must be familiar with your clinic's and your own symbolic value and establish coherence between what you are and what you communicate as a company.

"A salesperson who thinks that a lower price will sell more, does not know the symbolic value of things." *Jürgen Klarić*

An excessively low price can seem implausible to consumers. As a veterinary surgeon you work in health sciences, a sector where credibility, which is related to price, is vitally important. If your child is ill and you have two medicines, a very cheap product and a very expensive one from a well-known brand, which would you choose? There is an emotional bond that ensures we always want to give the best treatment to a sick child, and the best is associated with a higher price, whether we like it or not.

None of the world's leading brands are the cheapest in their sector. Yet there are brands that seem cheap, but they are not really, and others that have a very good price–quality relationship. However, the top brands are always expensive and never offer discounts.

Maybe your clinic will never become a world-renowned brand, but you could be a leading brand in your city or market niche.

9 Reception in a neuromarketing clinic

WINNING OVER THE SENSES. NEUROMARKETING AT THE RECEPTION

You can deliver better medicine by having an impact on emotions

In the first part of this chapter we will discuss how the reception is the physical access point to your practice and how the client's first impression enters through their sensory organs.

The second part will deal with the reception as a physical space, the client's arrival, and how they should be received.

Managing the waiting room as a customer care centre is essential for the economic success of your clinic.

As we have mentioned in previous chapters:

- The human being uses the emotional, and not just the rational, part of their brain to make decisions. In fact, between 85 % and 95 % of our decisions are made based on the indications of the emotional and primitive brain, the so-called reptilian brain. These are subconscious decisions.
- Feelings affect rationality; the logical part of the brain then justifies why we made the given decision.
- The aim is to seduce the client's brain and convert it into an ally, and this process transforms the act of purchasing into a pleasure. Can this be extrapolated to the dealings of a veterinary clinic?
- Generating pleasure increases client loyalty, which translates into repeat purchases.

People use shopping as a means of escape when feeling anxious, there are even cases of true addiction to brands or products. Can this be extrapolated to all sectors? How can we do it?

We know it takes less than 2.5 seconds to take a decision and make a value judgement. Just by passing the door of a restaurant we immediately create a mental image of the type of food, the menu, and the expected price range. The same thing happens to clients when they enter your veterinary practice.

Can a waiting room swing a client in favour or against a clinic? Apparently, yes it can.

Sensory organs: the first impression

As in life, the first impression your company emits is very important. What is a first impression? It is the first image or judgement we make about whatever is in front of us, an immediate reaction that decides between friend/enemy, like/dislike, or trust/distrust, for example. To a large extent this information is received through the sensory organs and subconsciously processed within seconds by the reptilian or primitive brain.

INTERESTING FACT

Depending on how each individual processes information, 40 % of people are more reliant on visual stimuli, another 40 % are kinaesthetic, that is, they predominantly use their sense of touch, smell, and taste, while the remaining 20 % are auditory.

Having said that, nobody is uniquely visual, auditory, or kinaesthetic, we all use a mixture of our senses but with a greater preference for one over the others. Let us look at how to recognise each type of client according to their sensory skills.

Kinaesthetic clients

Smell and taste

Human olfactory receptors are located in nasal epithelial cells. They are highly differentiated, which means each receptor can detect various odours before re-combining them to form a pattern.

Some odours and pheromones stimulate the hypothalamus and pituitary gland, for example those associated with sex, appetite, body temperature, or stress. In the neocortex, odours have an influence on long-term memory and can evoke memories. We have all smelt aromas that have brought back childhood recollections. Animals use pheromones as sexual attractants; pheromones also help them find their prey, identify rotten food, or detect and flee from an assailant.

Every home, person, city, and memory smells differently. The human being can distinguish up to 10,000 different odours, yet our sense of smell has gradually lost prominence over the course of evolution.

Only brands in specific sectors, such as the perfume, food, or bakery industries, have viewed aromas as an important strategic tool. Neuromarketing studies have shown that people can change their behaviour according to different scents.

Why is it so important to pay attention to odours in a veterinary clinic? What should a waiting room smell like? Is there a perfect or ideal scent?

When an agreeable experience is associated with a specific odour then it is stored in the person's memory. This also works in reverse, as odours can invoke a positive memory.

Brands try to trigger the same process in consumers. When a company forms an association in the consumer's mind between its brand and a given scent, then it is known as scent branding, which is part of the neurobranding concept. Certain products are connected to specific aromas. Some brands use their own scents: Audi works with their own aroma, Burger King uses the smell of grilled meat, and hotels such as The Cumberland or clothes shops employ their own perfumes.

The textile, food, and hospitality sectors currently employ the neurobranding concept. For example, in the case of clothing, an item's smell when the consumer gets home reminds them of the pleasurable purchasing event. The image of quality and prestige is linked to this olfactory experience.

Next is a list of some odours that have been studied in terms of neuromarketing and the impressions they induce in people:

- The smell of lemons or window cleaning products is associated with cleanliness.
- The smell of tobacco causes people to perceive spaces as being smaller.
- Floral and citric aromas encourage clients to spend more.

- The smell of pure alcohol or disinfectant is associated with hospitals.
- A metallic odour correlates with technology.
- Aromas such as vanilla, lavender, and chamomile promote a sense of relaxation. Vanilla is also associated with a sense of familiarity.
- Leather and cedar are used in fur retailers and offices because they invoke prestige.
- Regarding unpleasant smells, and which produce a negative mood, noteworthy odours are human sweat, raw onion, diarrhoea and faeces, decay, and rubbish in general.

When selling a house, for example, the scent of vanilla and coffee are known to increase sales. Shops that carry the scent of leather emit an image of quality and can charge higher prices.

However, you must be very careful with the intensity. A strong hospital smell can conjure up a bad memory of a previous hospital visit, thus losing the opportunity to create a good impression. In people with allergies or hypersensitivity reactions, an intense aroma could trigger rejection, not necessarily because of the odour, but because of a memory and the fear of the problem reappearing.

It is important to control the intensity of the fragrances you use in your clinic.

A scent is notable upon entering a room and lasts for 10 to 15 seconds, after which it fades away, as we can all remember from our years of practical classes at university.

Before selecting from a list of odours, we recommend you review the type of veterinary practice you are running, so you transmit a coherent message.

- If it is a family clinic, a vanilla aroma would be a good idea.
- In springtime, you could introduce citric or floral scents.
- If you own a small centre, a fresh aroma could make it feel more spacious.
- The toilets should smell clean or gel-like. If you are trying to create a hospital-like aspect, you should recreate the same odour.

The smell of dog, animal feed, excrement, or sweat are unacceptable in a 21st century clinic, so cleanliness is of the utmost importance in a veterinary centre. In fact, these tasks should be carried out by professional cleaners rather than the centre's vets or auxiliary staff. The first thing to use when faced with unpleasant smells are odour-neutralising products. You can then introduce the fragrances you have chosen for your clinic over this neutral odour.

You can combine different essences in the clinic's different rooms. However, you should not mix intense scents to avoid an overwhelming aroma; it is better to work on a common footing.

Essences are often oil-based and released as mists or allowed to evaporate from small bottles, they can even be incorporated into the clinic's ventilation system.

Taking a look at shopping centres, you will notice the aromas change throughout the day; for example, in the morning the cafeteria smells of baking and coffee roasting, while at lunchtime it smells of cooked food. These scents encourage people

Using scents around the clinic

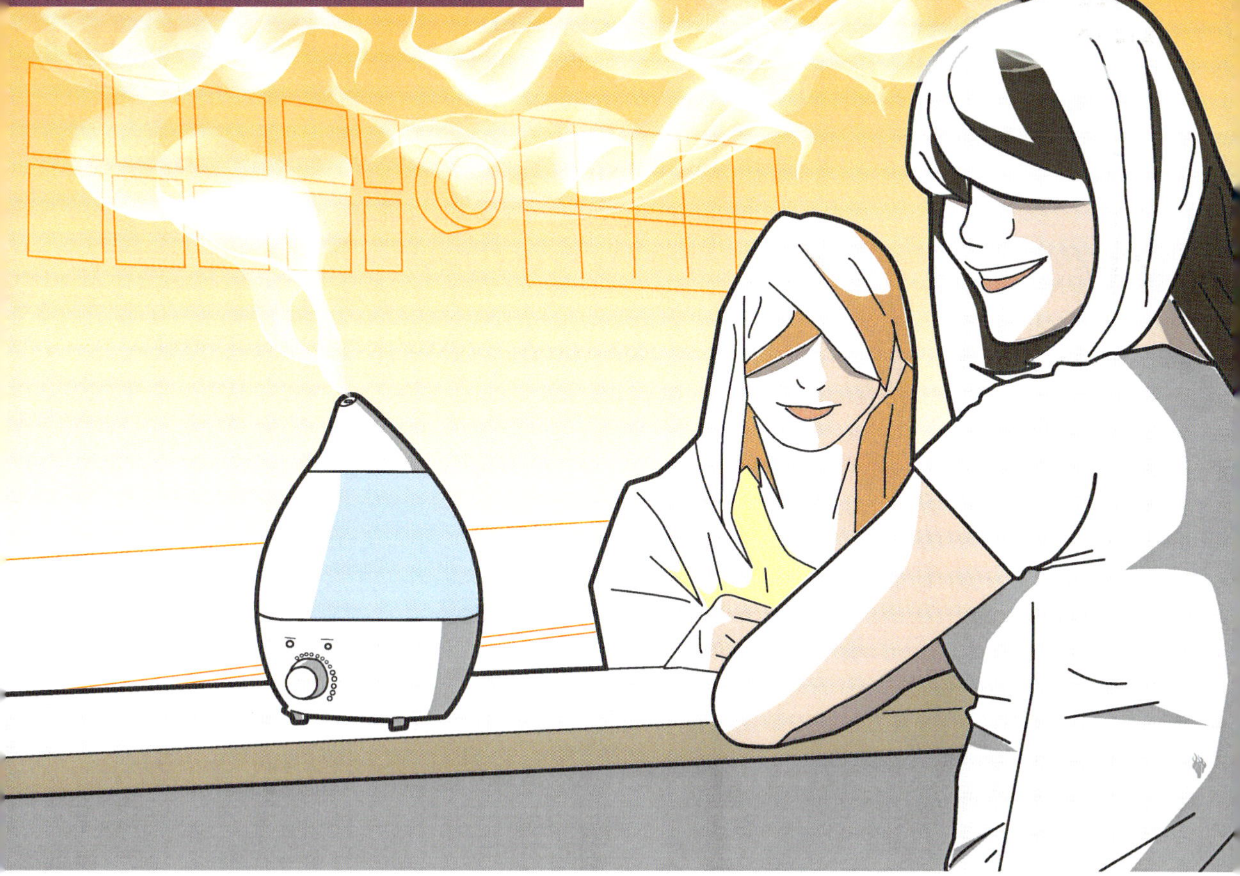

to consume. Venting the smell of bread outside a bakery or chocolate outside a chocolate shop helps increase the number of visitors.

We suggest you perfume the desk next to the cash register. Use aromas, scented candles, and essential oils that persuade people to enter, as the cash register is often close to the door. Studies conducted by Ikea have found that people remain in perfumed areas for 54 % longer, customer satisfaction increases by 7 %, and sales go up by 6 % when the atmosphere is filled with a pleasant aroma.

Touch

Our hands can recognise and perceive many different sensations, from temperature, roughness, cleanliness, to the quality of an object. Neuromarketing has shown that when purchasing electronic devices, remote controls, cameras, or telephones, we associate the weight of the object with a perception of superior quality and therefore a higher price. Drivers talk about the feeling of sitting in a car and stroking the steering wheel, which is a very important part of the purchasing process.

It is important to remember the role hands play in communication, expressivity, art, or intimacy; they are essential in nonverbal language and human communication.

Communicating written information on premium, heavyweight paper gives the information a sense of quality and trustworthiness. When selecting the type of paper used to print out a curriculum vitae, its weight bears an influence on the impression the candidate creates. Therefore, printed advertising sometimes uses high-quality paper and materials, as touching something with a pleasant feel stimulates oxytocin, a hormone associated with wellbeing.

You should pay attention to some very subtle aspects related to the sense of touch upon entering your clinic, for example, the quality of the door handles and knobs, or dust on packets of feed and other products, which will make them feel old or out of date. You must also focus on the feel of the reception counter, which must be pristine, or the towels in the toilets, which must be clean, and general tidiness.

The client will establish a direct association between what they see in reception and a company's unseen inner workings, and, in turn, the level of veterinary medicine practised at the centre. For example, if the waiting room is dirty, what will the operating room be like, especially considering it is out of sight?

If you want to achieve a sensation of quality in the waiting room, you should furnish it with high-quality, comfortable seats. To appear meticulous, the magazines must be recent and in good condition, there should be no sticky surfaces, and any leaflets the clients touch must be orderly and dust free.

It is important consumers can always touch any products you offer them.

EXAMPLE

Don't just talk about a diet, hand the package to the customer, so their level of acceptance increases upon touching it. As such, you should place small, tangible objects near the cash register. The fact they can see and hold them increases the possibility of acceptance and an impulsive purchase. Small items, for instance, treats, collars, and the like, must be within the consumer's reach. The most important point regarding this type of purchase is the ability to grasp the object, weigh it up, turn it around, and view it in 3D; in the case of pet food, clients tend to read the product information and ingredients only after touching and feeling the package. To be precise, this is termed instrumental information.

Still, the act of touching and the sensory experience when feeling an object is more hedonistic than we think, as occurs with fluffy towels or woollen jumpers; this also applies to puppies, which we hug and smell to obtain a more complete and pleasurable experience. This purchasing pattern is essential for one type of consumer, so they prefer not to buy things on the internet as it eliminates this pleasure.

Touch is strongly linked to the packaging and the aspect of conceptualising a brand.

The type of packaging, paper, and even the weight of the packet can give an impression of roughness, mass, or toughness that could lead to the product being rejected. So, feed packets should be smooth to the touch and easy to handle. Quality packaging means customers perceive quality contents. This is apparent in the bottled water market, where glass bottles are associated with better quality.

Touch is directly related to expressiveness. Gesticulation serves to reinforce language. If you are establishing a possible diagnosis, then avoid putting your hands in your pockets, scratching an ear, or touching your hair or face as these gestures reflect doubt. To strengthen a message, show the palms of your open hands as this bolsters the credibility of your words.

Studies have shown that:

- The sense of touch is closely linked to empathy.
  - Shaking hands or touching the client or patient creates a sense of closeness and good manners, so be sure not to undervalue this contact. By the same token, putting your hand on the client's shoulder or arm at a painful time produces a feeling of understanding and support. Greeting owners correctly in reception and shaking hands or stroking the dog and calling them by their name are essential for building trust.
- The sense of touch influences feelings and behaviour.
  - Neuromarketing discusses the haptic experience, which involves the study of feelings and behaviour in connection with touch. In sales they would talk about the feeling when touching an object and the pleasure generated by this sense. If accompanied by a story, the brain triggers the release of oxytocin which is associated with shopping and pleasure. These feelings generate the need to repeat the pleasurable experience, thereby creating brand loyalty. A hand stretching out through a window during a car advert conjures up an image of flying. It is therefore important to consider images and touch as a means of producing feelings and a connection to a purchase. In the veterinary industry, this sense is used in adverts with adorable puppies that whimper or lick their owners while being hugged. Likewise, if any member of your team hugs a puppy it shows that your clinic loves animals and you send a very clear message to the owner.

Visual clients

Colours and emotional codes

Visible light is the narrow range of electromagnetic radiation encompassing wavelengths of 380 to 760 nanometres; lower values include infrared and microwave radiation, whereas ultraviolet light is found above the visible range.

Each species perceives light differently; cats can see at much weaker light intensities than humans, while insects and birds can see ultraviolet light. On the other hand, many mammals do not discern between many different colours, but they can distinguish a lot of smells. However, we are still not completely sure how animals see.

Throughout evolution, human beings have always shown a great deal of interest in colours. In the Middle Ages, a large industry grew around trading in scale insect dyes or silks. Different cultures have developed relationships with and codes involving colours, using them in ceremonies or staining their bodies or hair.

The cone cells in the human retina react to white light. These cells detect red, green, and blue wavelengths. Hence, human vision is said to be trichromatic, that is, we see in red, green, and blue, which are of course the primary colours of light (RGB).

Each human eye receives information individually and in two dimensions, in other words, one eye on its own cannot appreciate depth of field. The visual cortex, located in the prefrontal cortex of the brain, interprets this information and transforms it into a three-dimensional image. Colours and shading help the visual cortex decipher shapes and recognise objects. Upon entering a room, the eyes perform a visual sweep or quick examination by looking straight ahead and then to the right. The tendency is to progressively increase the peripheral field of vision. Therefore, it is very important that your reception has a place to head for upon entering, such as a counter, as it orients the client and makes them feel secure.

Colours take on a different meaning in different cultures; the colour of mourning is black in some areas and white in others. The emotions people develop in association with a colour depends on their life experiences, for example, someone forced to wear navy blue when they were a child may detest it as an adult.

The following generalisations apply to emotions stimulated by colours:

- Yellow improves mood. The eye recognises it quickly and it emits a feeling of "newness". It can also represent precaution.

- Orange is arousing, but if it is very bright it may cause nervousness. It is also related to power, youthfulness, and healthy eating. In addition, orange is a very eye-catching colour.
- Red is very dynamic and energetic, it is used by a lot of drinks. In veterinary medicine, it could be connected to blood, so it should be used cautiously, in faint touches or strokes, rather than to cover entire walls, for example. On the other hand, in Asian cultures, such as Chinese, Japanese, and Korean cultures, red is associated with good luck, success, and the start of a new year or cycle. Laying out red fruits in restaurants is known to entice diners to order more food.
- Pink induces friendliness and, in certain cultures, is related to childhood and the female sex.
- White creates clarity in the ambiance and in people's thoughts. White clothes are linked to wisdom and experience. It is a suitable colour for gowns, but they must be spotlessly clean and perfectly ironed. Rooms painted white appear larger. It is also associated with purity and cleanliness.
- Brown leather or wood in interior decorations gives an impression of quality. A packet of coffee packaged in shades of brown produces an image of having a strong flavour and intense aroma.
- Black is affiliated to mystery, sophistication, power, and authority. It works very well for cars but not airplanes. It is also associated with mourning and death.
- Precious metal colours, such as gold, silver, or platinum, bear a relation to a high price, wealth, and status. They are used in the perfume and cosmetic sectors because they create a feeling of belonging to a prestigious group. Similarly, these colours are popular in Russia and the Middle East where they represent power and grandeur.
- Blue is a calm, relaxing colour that inspires respect and authority. It has the least intercultural variation across Asia, Africa, and Europe. It stimulates respect, but also gentleness, depending on the format and product in question; baby clothes or coffee in blue packaging would be regarded as mild. Additionally, blue is also linked to purity, as can be seen in the mineral water market or the religious sector.
- Green is associated with nature. It is relaxing, friendly, and natural. It is linked to a good working atmosphere, ecology, and the environment.

You must decide if you want to establish a mental association in your client's mind that connects your business to the medical sector. If your centre is a large veterinary hospital, it may be more appropriate to use colours associated with human medicine, such as white, green, or blue, while elements such as gowns and uniforms should tie in with this concept.

Colours

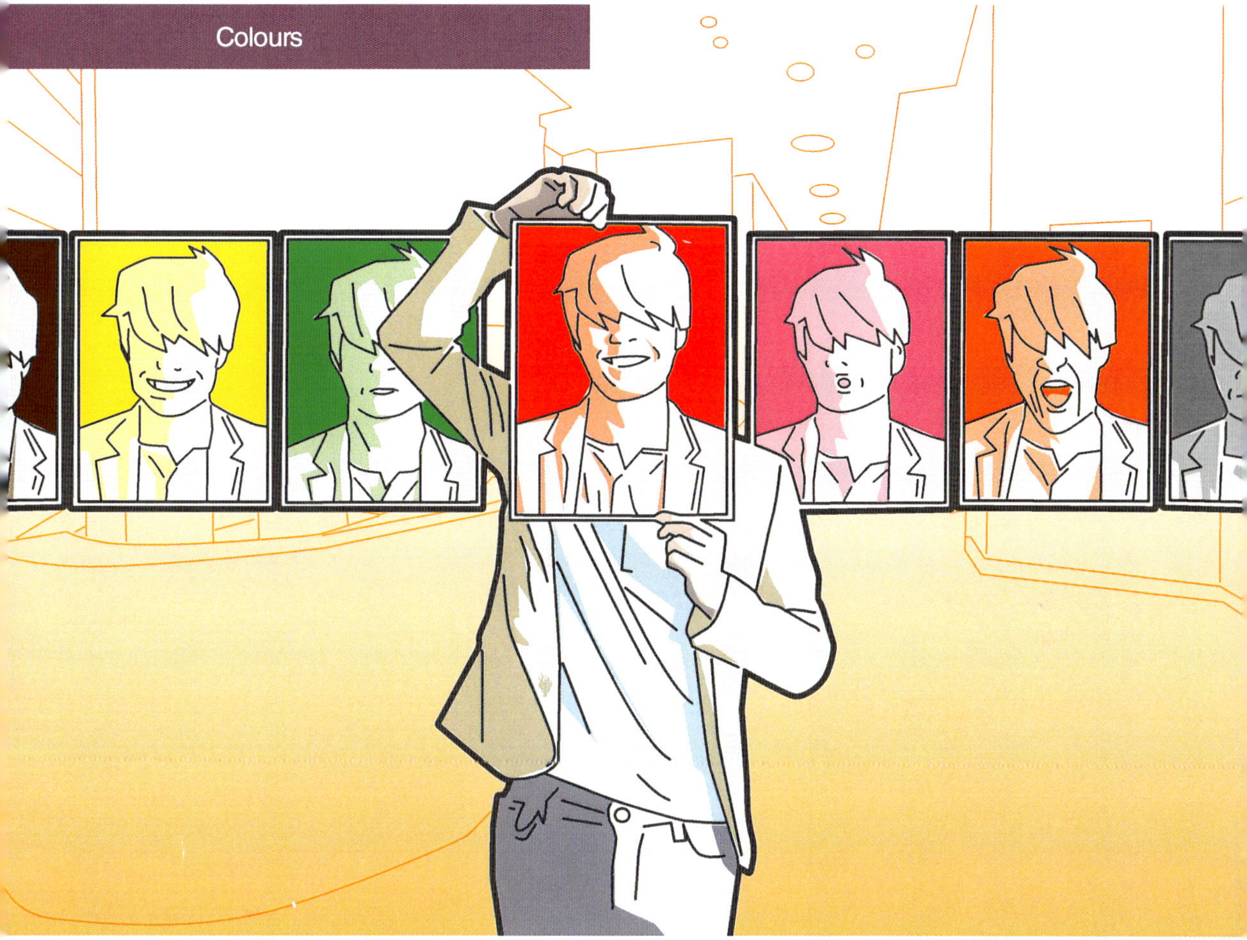

You also need to think about the colours you will use for your clinic's logo and advertisements. As underlined when discussing coherence, you must remember if the waiting room is one colour, the uniforms must match, as should logos and advertising. One form of coherence is to select colour codes and use them in the different settings.

In theory, associations are neither good nor bad, but in children a white or green gown may be associated with a stressful situation experienced in a hospital or a negative medical event. That is why there are no magic formulae, although you must consider the type of service you offer when deciding.

If you own a close, friendly clinic, you have more room to manoeuvre when selecting gowns and colours, this is also true if the clinic's staff are quite young. Nevertheless, the centre's entire decoration and ambiance must follow the same lines.

The colour code also emanates information about sturdiness, agility, or aspects such as strength and durability. In the household appliances market, statistically, if a man is purchasing a vacuum cleaner he will tend to select black and red models because they appear to be more robust, while a woman is more likely to choose models in lighter shades because they perceive them as easier to use or lightweight. The same thing happens with cars, or in the case of cranes where yellow or red are firmly implanted.

Colours selected for veterinary practices tend to radiate experience and reliability, but with a touch of closeness.

White, green, and blue shades are a safe option, and should be mixed with furniture featuring wooden or metallic tones, in step with your personality.

Another point worth highlighting relates to the intensity of chrome-coloured furniture; brighter or more saturated colours are known to lift people's mood.

INTERESTING FACT

There is an area of the brain, the PTO, located between the parietal, temporal, and occipital lobes, where visual information is combined with our sense of touch, hearing, and smell. Each person's image of a dog, for example, is assembled here by combining information about smell, shape, characteristic sound (barking), and touch. Hence, we talk about multifactorial perception.

Senses such as smell and touch disappear when browsing through the "e-landscape" known as the internet, so colours and the way they are distributed across the screen predominate. Studies have found that internet users seek consistency between the music and colour scheme of the sites they visit, plus the human eye is attracted by movement. It is interesting to know that our gaze is drawn by the location where others are looking. If a model is looking at a poster, we will also look at it. Therefore, you must consider eye movement to be equally decisive as colours when it comes to browsing the internet.

Google now features an option to set up virtual tours of veterinary practices, in which case all these colour codes will assume even greater importance when trying to build client loyalty and invite them to visit your clinic in person. Neuromarketing is implemented with the aid of new technologies such as eye tracking.

Auditory clients

Music, tone of voice, sounds, language

Sound is vibration, and the human ear can detect frequencies ranging from 20 to 200,000 hertz. Just as with sight we were interested in visible light, here we are interested in audible sounds. Ranges of sound perception vary between species.

One of the most significant differences between humans and animals is that of musical creativity. In evolutionary terms, we do not know why human beings felt they needed to start making music. In anthropological terms, it can be linked to a social connection between group members, as all cultures manifest the ability to create music. There are various theories concerning musical creativity, but one of them suggests that the development of certain brain functions opened a door for the expression of music, art, and dance.

Music is processed in the brain, not only as an audible experience, but also as a motor event, because it activates areas associated with dance and movement. It also generates feelings and evokes memories. Long-term memory connected to childhood means we all develop a musical memory.

It is important to consider the strength of sounds and be able to differentiate between noises (both pleasant and unpleasant) and the music you want to play in reception.

Neuromarketing studies the impact of music at the points where you interact with clients, and how it can awaken memories and experiences in a very personal manner. The table that follows cites a series of recommendations you could implement in your veterinary business.

We can talk about brand-related music, for example large chains repeatedly play their slogan or theme song interlaced with the background music. Enjoyment derived from music can increase consumption.

TIPS FOR SELECTING MUSIC IN YOUR VETERINARY PRACTICE

Music should be instrumental, so that people can still concentrate on conversations.

It should not be raucous, but rather quite neutral.

The volume of music affects enthusiasm and mood.

In certain settings, music is strongly linked to traditions; therefore, regional or Christmas music should be saved for specific periods of the year, particularly if they are connected to presents and consumption.

Cheerful music produces happiness; sad music, anxiety; and repetitive music causes boredom and nervousness.

How and when should I play music in my veterinary practice?

1. In the waiting room. It could be neutral music. You should bear in mind your clinic type, in the same way as with the colour scheme and decoration. If the waiting room is upmarket, you could play classical, jazz, or new age music. In a more youthful waiting room, pop music might be more appropriate with something lighter at midday.

2. In the treatment room. As music could reduce the client's concentration, we recommend neutral music at a low volume, piped music, or none whatsoever.

3. If you sedate the animal in the client's presence, you could play relaxing music to soothe the owner's stress.

4. Avoid rap or rock music if you want to concentrate and create a pleasant atmosphere.

5. At the point of sale. Play soft music at a low volume as it will have a positive influence at the point of sale.

6. During staff meetings, administrative tasks, or in the laboratory. Music has been shown to improve the working atmosphere and make work a more pleasant experience.

Music and ambient

Musical rhythm is known to affect movement above all. Therefore, in a commercial space, fast-paced music accelerates the passage of consumers, thus affecting the time they spend in the store, even without the customer realising. This occurs even in people who are not consciously listening to the music. Clothes shops for young people play radio format music so the public imagines themselves in a club-like setting. We do not know why exactly, but actions such as walking, moving around, or talking tend to match a background rhythm.

The important point is that music creates an ambiance, changes mood, and conveys and evokes memories. It is also associated with a lifestyle, so you can use it to address a target audience.

When entering a waiting room, the ambient sound is not only related to the musical selection but also to the noises that can be heard at that given moment. Unpleasant sounds, such as children shouting or a barking dog, produce stress and a bad impression upon entry.

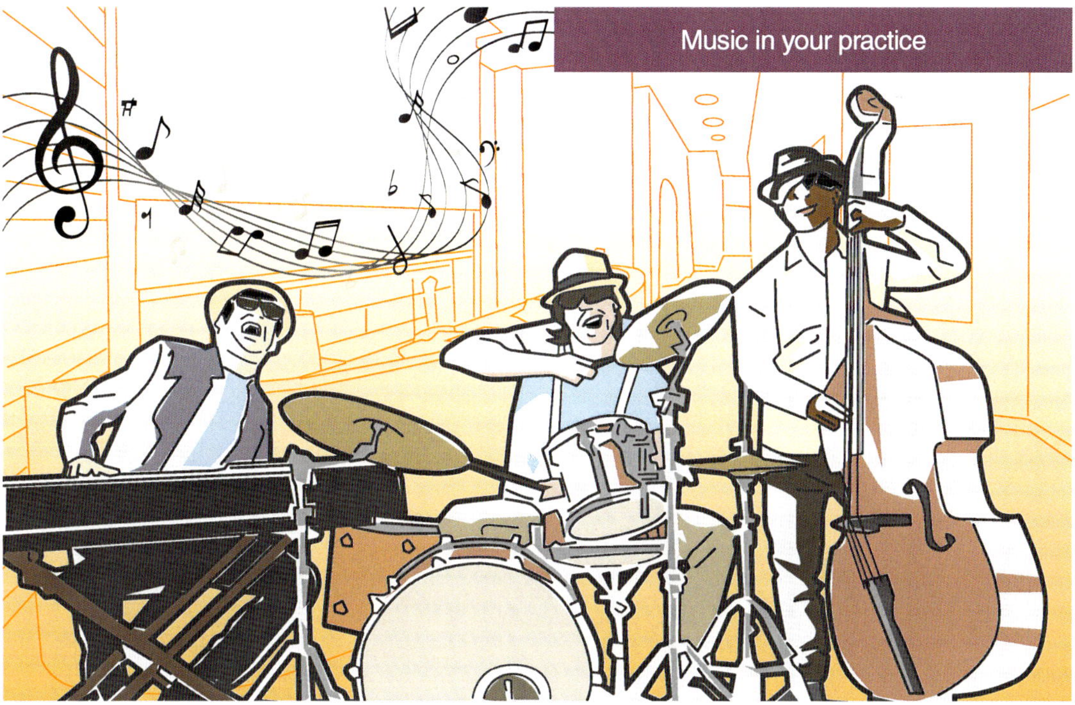

Voice

The first thing a client looks for when entering the reception is the person who will attend them. It is confusing, and raises doubts, when a client finds themselves in an empty reception.

The client must know where to turn when they enter the reception; people feel uncomfortable if they enter the clinic and are confronted by an empty counter.

In the same vein, it is extremely important that the person staffing reception applies the following skills and practices. The receptionist should

- Greet the person who has just entered with a smile.
- Ask them how they can help.
- Recognise the owner and pet or record their contact details correctly if it is the first time the client has visited the veterinary centre.
- Reward and greet the pet as well.
- Say something positive about the animal.
- Be polite and pleasant, and it is vital that they express themselves and address others naturally and consistently.
- Look straight at clients and reflect genuine interest, suspending any other activities which could make the client feel they are not receiving their full attention.

A well-positioned business, with fitting design and decoration, and carefully thought-out sensory characteristics may be insufficient if you do not look after reception correctly, because people and how they behave are the most important feature of communication.

The waiting room as a point of contact

To make the waiting room more profitable you must address some communication-related aspects: close out sales, arrange the next appointment, present information about health plans and any offers on products and services, manage payments, and, of course, create an excellent first impression.

IMPORTANT DETAILS IN THE WAITING ROOM

If the client has to wait to be attended after entering the clinic, you could give them a task to complete at reception, such as filling out and checking their file, or completing some information about the reason for their pet's consultation. This will help the vet greet the client and patient and get them up to speed on the reason for their visit. Additionally, being accompanied and helped to fill out a form reduces the waiting sensation for the owner.

You must take special care when drafting this brief form. Use it to discover whether the owner was referred by another client or found your clinic on the internet. Learning about any other animals they may have owned in the past will help establish a trust-based relationship. The vet must receive this information and read it before starting the consultation, the client should not have to repeat the entire history.

You must help people with a degree of disability. Your customers will include elderly people who cannot stand while waiting and need somewhere to sit down. The waiting room should have up-to-date magazines or reading material, or an application connected to a screen to provide information about your services and present pet-based news stories.

Ensure the magazines do not contain unpleasant images or content more appropriate for veterinary professionals, although they can feature news items and educational pieces about the animal world.

The receptionist should inform clients in the waiting room about any incidents, for example, if their appointment is going to be delayed or if an emergency has arisen. Give them an indication about how much longer they will have to wait and thank them for their understanding.

Placing products within reach or sight, if they are heavy, will encourage more impulse purchases in the waiting area. Products with the highest rotation can generally be placed in the least visible location, while you should position those you want to promote at eye level. If you recommend a product, it is a good idea to let the client touch it, because this helps project it into their mind, so they can imagine themselves owning the item. Visual clients will hardly listen to technical information, whereas auditory ones like to hear this data. When giving information about pet diets to a visual client, it is better to use expressions such as, "Bobby will grow strong and avoid nutritional problems", rather than talk about protein content, as clients find it easier to visualise stories in their minds, especially if they carry an emotional load.

Listening

A good salesperson listens before speaking and directs the conversation to the speaker's necessities. We have two ears and just one mouth.

You must develop your sense of listening to become a better salesperson. If you know the client's needs, you can offer them the right products and services and sell the advantages to them.

- If the client talks about their family or children, they are more likely to buy a specific diet if we recommend it by highlighting that their "dog will produce more solid stools that are easier to collect" or "will grow stronger and develop fewer illnesses".
- If the owner mentions they train with their pet and go running every afternoon, you should stress that a specific diet will give their animal more energy and make them stronger.
- Recommendations regarding deworming and flea and tick treatments should focus on the benefits of keeping the client's pet healthy and preventing disease transmission to the family and children. To this end, it is a good idea to base your narrative around real events, so the listener can put themselves in the shoes of these other clients and decide if they want to run the same risk. It is better to

work with stories rather than hard facts since they influence the reptilian brain, which is the area that looks after the family's safety.

- When the client leaves the consulting room, the auxiliary staff must check they are satisfied and have noted the next appointment in their agenda, with the specific time and date, even if it is not for another 6 months. We recommend asking them if they wish to receive a reminder by phone, text, email, WhatsApp, or Facebook as it demonstrates your commitment to the client. After setting up the contact method for the reminder, explain when you will get in touch with the client or how you will manage their pet's follow-up. It is preferable that staff at your clinic take the initiative as opposed to leaving it for the client to arrange the next appointment. This option is left for those who do not know their shifts and working hours far enough in advance.
- You should ask if the pet owner has understood all the information or if they have any questions, as they often fail to absorb everything they are told during the consultation due to nerves. It is very helpful if the vet hands the client a short written report during the appointment, including any recommendations and prescribed treatments.
- You must train auxiliary staff so they can give a clear explanation of the vet's note and immediately correct any errors they may notice.
- Although we will discuss the payment stage later, from a neuromarketing perspective it is one of the most important moments during a visit as the client has to let go of something. It is crucial to generate pleasure at this point in order to minimise the pain associated with the loss. Eating small portions of chocolate when paying is known to reduce this pain, as does a pleasant aroma in the payment area.
- Congratulate the owner for using your services because an early diagnosis always results in a quicker resolution with less impact for their pet. If you say something like, "*Shep* is so lucky to have an owner like you", it will create a feeling of belonging and care, while minimising any unease concerning the expense. It is the same feeling you get when you buy a shirt, if the sales assistant says something nice about the colour while folding it, or how exclusive it is, how much it will suit you, or that they have a similar one. This feeling generates pleasure and a long-term memory, and it works the brand into the client's mind.
- This a good opportunity to reiterate how committed you are and that the client can call to discuss any doubts with the vet who is handling their pet, thereby attaching added value to the payment they are making.
- It is also a good time to confirm that you have their correct contact details, in case someone from the clinic wants to check on the patient's progress.
- Finally, owners appreciate any courtesy shown when they are leaving, as they may often need help carrying their pet to the car or, at the very least, you should accompany them to the door and hold it open for them. This means your staff must show willingness and a client-friendly service attitude.

POINTS TO REMEMBER

- When a client arrives at your practice, the first thing they physically interact with is the reception and waiting room. All the decorative and sensory details should give off an accurate impression of what they will find in the clinic. Odours, colours, staff uniforms, furniture, and the attitude and behaviour of the entire team must be in harmony, so the client perceives a coherent message. You only get one chance to create a good first impression.
- Employ active listening to obtain all the information required to make the veterinary surgeon's job easier so that the client feels confident and you can exceed their expectations.
- Creating a pleasant atmosphere when it is time to pay, to arrange the next appointment, and to say goodbye, will help ensure the client returns to your clinic.

10 Conquering your client's mind. Neuromarketing in the consultation room

Basic communication considerations

The consultation room is your "centre of operations", the scene where veterinary surgeons and pets take centre stage. Hence the importance of value generation based on a communication and language approach. Both aspects build confidence, and this helps clients accept estimates for necessary veterinary procedures.

You should construct the path for the client to follow in your veterinary practice. They will have previously assessed the attention they received on the telephone when making an appointment, the ease of parking near the clinic, and the ease of access to the clinic if they have a disability, for example. Once inside, the reception staff fulfil a vital role as they represent the company's cover letter.

When the pet owner goes from the waiting room to the consultation room, the first thing they encounter is the veterinary surgeon. We are not going to dwell on the odours and other factors that have an impact on the senses during this first impression, but it is advisable to reflect on the image you portray to others, just as you would when meeting a human healthcare professional.

In light of the pet humanisation process that is sweeping across the world, our work as vets is becoming comparable to that of a paediatrician. When a client's pet is ill, they experience a level of stress similar to that of a parent whose child is unwell.

What is more, the low fertility rates in Western society mean pets are often the babies of the household and are considered one of the family along with the children.

If you have children, think about the type of medical care you would like them to receive and this will tell you what a client expects from you as their vet. Appearance, empathy, professionalism, friendliness, courtesy, and the right words at the right time, are essential elements to which you must pay the utmost attention as a professional. The client will judge you according to their standards and these are usually the points that will tip the balance in your favour when trying to win their trust.

External image

Several details have a direct effect on the professional image you emanate with your first impression:

1. Personal hygiene
   - This has a direct impact on the client's mind, as they will associate it with the type of veterinary medicine you practice, so it is always a good idea to check yourself in the mirror before entering the consultation room. Some veterinary clinics install mirrors next to the entrance of the consultation rooms.
   - In mixed clinics, which treat both large and small animals, veterinary surgeons often arrive from working in the countryside, put on their gowns, and get straight to work. Access to a shower is an important detail to consider and it only takes 10 minutes. The impression created by sweat or tobacco, for example, can have a stronger influence on the primitive mind than good veterinary care.
   - You should also pay attention to oral hygiene and the cleanliness of your hands. It would be like visiting the dentist and noticing they have an unhealthy mouth. How can you recommend dental prophylaxis for pets if you don't look after your own oral hygiene?
2. White gown
   - The Milgram experiment on obedience to authority figures was conducted after the Second World War and in the context of Nazi war crime trials. The study analysed the effects of uniforms and gowns on factors related to authority, as many soldiers sheltered behind the excuse that they were following orders and therefore absolved of responsibility for their actions.
   - The truth is that a certain type of clothing is associated with the concept of authority. This is evidenced by tribal and religious ceremonies, or music and political events in both Western and tribal societies.
   - The client assesses the veterinary surgeon based on the principle of authority. So you must be careful about any comments or opinions you express during a consultation. In addition, if the client bases decisions according to the principle of authority, there is no doubt that any failures will always be the vet's responsibility.
   - Neuromarketing in sales and hospitality industries continually makes use of uniforms to subconsciously let people know there is a chain of command and the level of authority they are dealing with. This is most apparent in the armed services and religious organisations. Brands use this tool in both chain stores and healthcare, as uniforms reinforce the image and quality of the brand and bear an influence of up to 30 % on the initial success and the positive impact on the client's brain.

- It is worth remembering that white gowns must be spotless and perfectly ironed; a gown stained with blood or faeces, for instance, would rapidly deface the very image you are working to create.

3. **The combination of a gown and stethoscope hung around your neck** will improve your credibility and success.
4. **ID cards with names and job titles** will increase the owner's level of trust because they know who they are talking to.

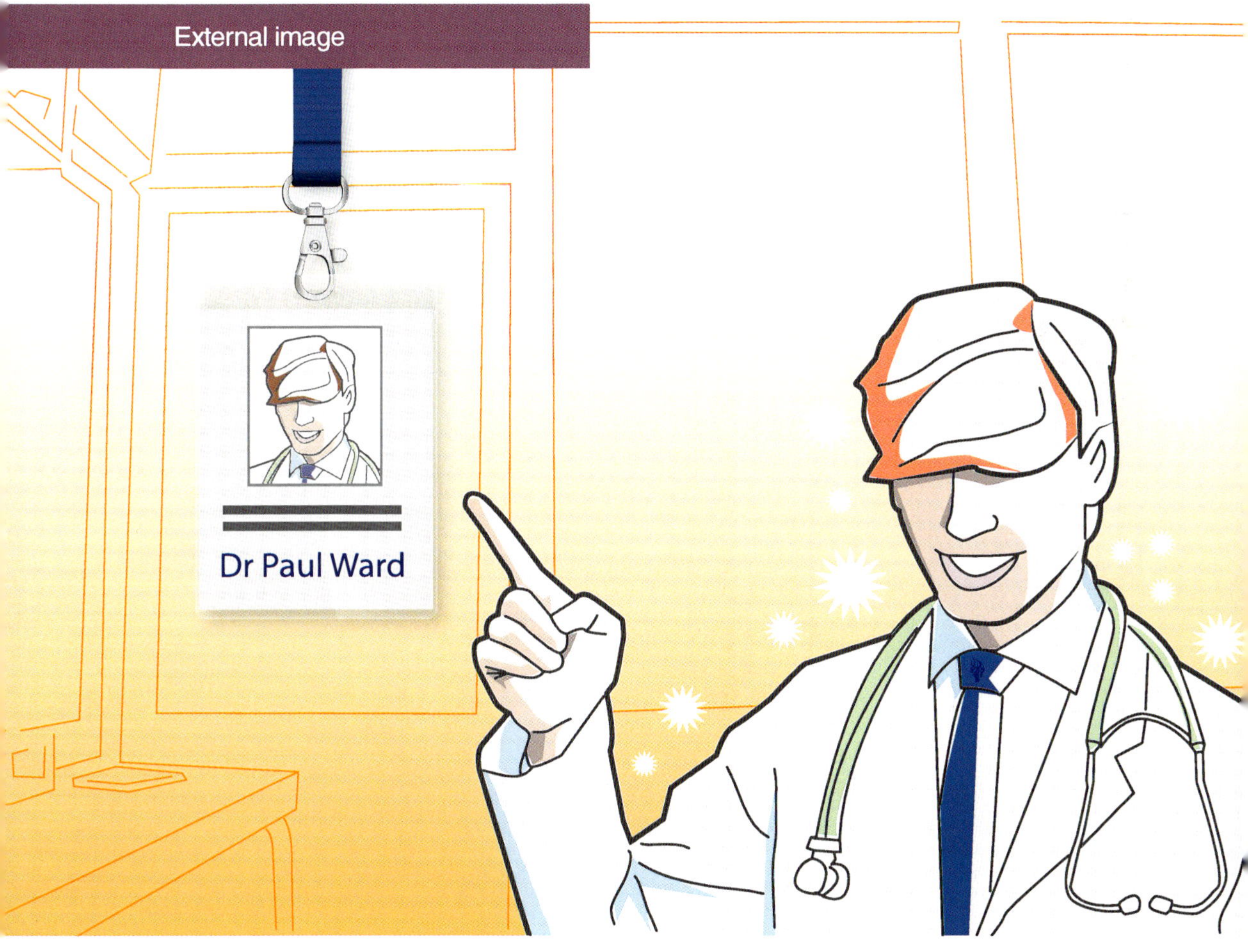

THE MILGRAM EXPERIMENT

A uniformed monitor ordered people, who believed they were helping conduct an experiment on memory and learning, to inflict punishments in the form of electric shocks on the "learners" (who were actually actors). Over 50 % of the participants inflicted the punishments up to limits that could have killed the "learners" (people they didn't even know), had these really received the electric shocks. Interestingly enough, when conducted today, the experiment still produces similar results.

Gestural image and emotions

Facial communication is very powerful for human beings. The primitive brain always tries to find an ally, so the client's gaze tends to focus on the vet's face. The most important detail is an honest, broad smile. The perfect smile would create those little wrinkles around your eyes known as laugh lines, because the decision-making brain picks up on forced smiles which lack smiling eyes and classifies them as false, thus creating mistrust due to the incoherence between the different areas of the face.

Neuromarketing has identified six basic emotions, each linked to its own facial expression, and you need to learn how to work with them. The crucial point is that these basic emotions fix events in people's memories. You must learn to recognise them in the speaker's face, so you can act accordingly, and how to consciously control them in your own face.

There are other emotions that feature their own facial language: confusion, pride, elevation, interest, and gratitude. It is better to deal with this group of emotions at the end of consultations, as they also induce pleasure and a desire to repeat the purchasing process.

Basic emotions

Happiness	From a neuromarketing perspective, you will achieve more sales and have more estimates accepted when your clients are happy. There are various situations when clients feel very cheerful in the veterinary clinic, perhaps the most obvious being when they arrive with a new puppy. At this moment, they are much more likely to accept a full vaccination plan including deworming, flea and tick treatments and regular checkups. People consume more when they are glad and euphoric, as happiness is associated with joy and a lack of fear; it is linked to pleasure and pleasure generates consumption. You can easily recognise happiness in the client's facial expression, it is associated with a smile, raised eyebrows, and an uplifted face.
Surprise	If you are pleasantly surprising, you will exceed your client's expectations and etch yourself into their memory. In the veterinary clinic, you should use a lot of phrases connected to emotions. For example, phrases such as "Don't worry the analysis will be ready in 10 minutes", or "The injection doesn't hurt and only takes a moment"; or simply inciting the animal to constantly greet all your staff so that the owner feels at home. Surprise is associated with enlarged eyes, an open mouth, and a slight inhalation.
Sadness	When connected to significant events, sadness creates a long-term memory and fear. It is also strongly linked to affection, so you must handle it very carefully when dealing with delicate subjects such as death, pain, or terminal illness.
Anger or irritation	This is related to conquering the opponent. When the client is angry, neuromarketing recommends you give them time to vent their frustration, until you see their facial expression change. We will discuss this in the section on handling complaints.
Aversion	This is associated with disgust and hygiene habits, as was discussed earlier.
Fear	Fear is almost worthy of its own chapter, because it is one of the feelings that creates the most strongly bound memories as they are deeply implanted in our brains and in those of animals. There is a range of different responses to fear and as a vet you may encounter them during consultations. When dealing with patients, some are fearful, while others are happy, but there are also those for whom a visit to the vet may induce an aggressive response. Fear originates in the amygdala and its influence over people can directly inhibit their thought and decision-making processes. So you must avoid reinforcing any fears when presenting an estimate or different treatment options to ensure the client's decision-making brain is not paralysed, thus enabling them to take a decision. It is much more effective if you underline the positive interpretations and let the client know there is a plausible path and outcome open to them. Humans experience two main types of fear: uncertainty and ridicule. ■ Fear of uncertainty: the brain does not want to confront complex risks; therefore, it locks up when faced with a dilemma or difficult decision. ■ Fear of ridicule: this is connected to the fear of criticism or feeling foolish.

We have already discussed image and how to read the client's mood, but we should also highlight the importance of mirror neurons, which help us make these readings and empathise. Empathy not only allows us to appreciate how someone else feels, it also activates an imitation mechanism. For example, when talking to someone who is euphoric, we tend to move our hands more or match our tone of voice with theirs. Mirror neurons assist us with our social skills. Being aware of this point helps when trying to shape a person's mood, so they find it easier to decide.

Practical application in the veterinary clinic

An important element of your work as a veterinary surgeon is selling intangibles. This means that the perceived value of your veterinary consultations is not based on the sale of products or prescription of medicines, but rather on a series of decisions you make regarding your patients' health, which are founded on your scientific knowledge.

The client's brain will make judgements in accordance with their own criteria, so they cannot evaluate your veterinary interventions unless they are healthcare professionals, but they will have an opinion about how a scar heals, how much interest you show in your patients, or the way you communicate.

You must learn to transform the intangible into something tangible by verbalising and explaining what you are doing.

An owner's connection to their pet is through the right side of their brain, whereas they associate with their vet through the left, which is the rational side. Initially you should relate with the emotional, right-hand side to establish a bond, then switch to the left side of their brain, which deals with logic and reasoning.

When your clients enter the consultation room, greet them using both the owner's and pet's name. In the example that follows, the animal is called Bobby. Ask why Bobby has come to see you and what is worrying his owner, Mrs Campbell. Ensure you do not stray from the central focus; concentrate on the reason why the animal is there.

Perhaps the reason for consultation is a skin complaint but during examination you detect a more urgent problem affecting the patient's knee. As mentioned in previous chapters, in this situation you should never lose sight of the client's perspective; first resolve the reason for their visit, then invite them to make another appointment for the second problem.

While listening, you often have to process extra information. For example, if the owner tells you Bobby is vomiting, you start thinking about the complementary tests their pet requires. Regardless of whether or not you are listening, you must give the impression you are fully focused. How can you do this? How can the client perceive this, bearing in mind you still haven't lifted the animal onto the examination table?

- Firstly, nod your head and raise your eyebrows. Make an affirmative sound while nodding your head if you want to stress the importance of a specific point. In addition, tilting your head to one side also shows you are interested and the speaker will notice this interest.
- Avoid gestures indicative of nervousness, such as touching your face or hair, scratching an ear, or biting on a pen or your nails. These gestures imply doubt and create uncertainty about whatever you are communicating.
- Repeating what you have heard emphasises that you are listening actively. In the present example, it would be something like "Mrs Campbell, I understand Bobby has had diarrhoea for 2 days, and you're very worried because Charlie, your last dog, died following a similar episode."
- Wait until the client confirms this point and give them the chance to add something further, then nod again.
- Verbalisation is very important in this pre-exam exchange, in fact you should end this stage by saying something such as "Okay, let's get started with Bobby's physical examination." This is when you generate the tangible element of the veterinary consultation.
- After this period of active listening and repeating what you have been told, lift Bobby onto the table and start examining him. Explain what you are doing in each step of the examination, whether palpating his lymph nodes or abdomen, or examining his mucous membranes. This leads to the "stethoscope moment" when you should politely request silence.

The way we express ourselves varies between cultures, but all clients need to be heard and feel they are being listened to.

Why do we have to play out and verbalise our work? For us it may seem obvious that we've checked out Bobby's breathing and heart, for example, but studies have shown that when clients are later asked in the waiting room if their animal underwent a physical examination, a relatively high percentage say no.

You should describe the entire physical exam in words to give it the importance it deserves. Remember the owner is not a healthcare worker, so they do not know what you are doing – they just see you touching their animal, then handing them an invoice.

Clients in the consultation room

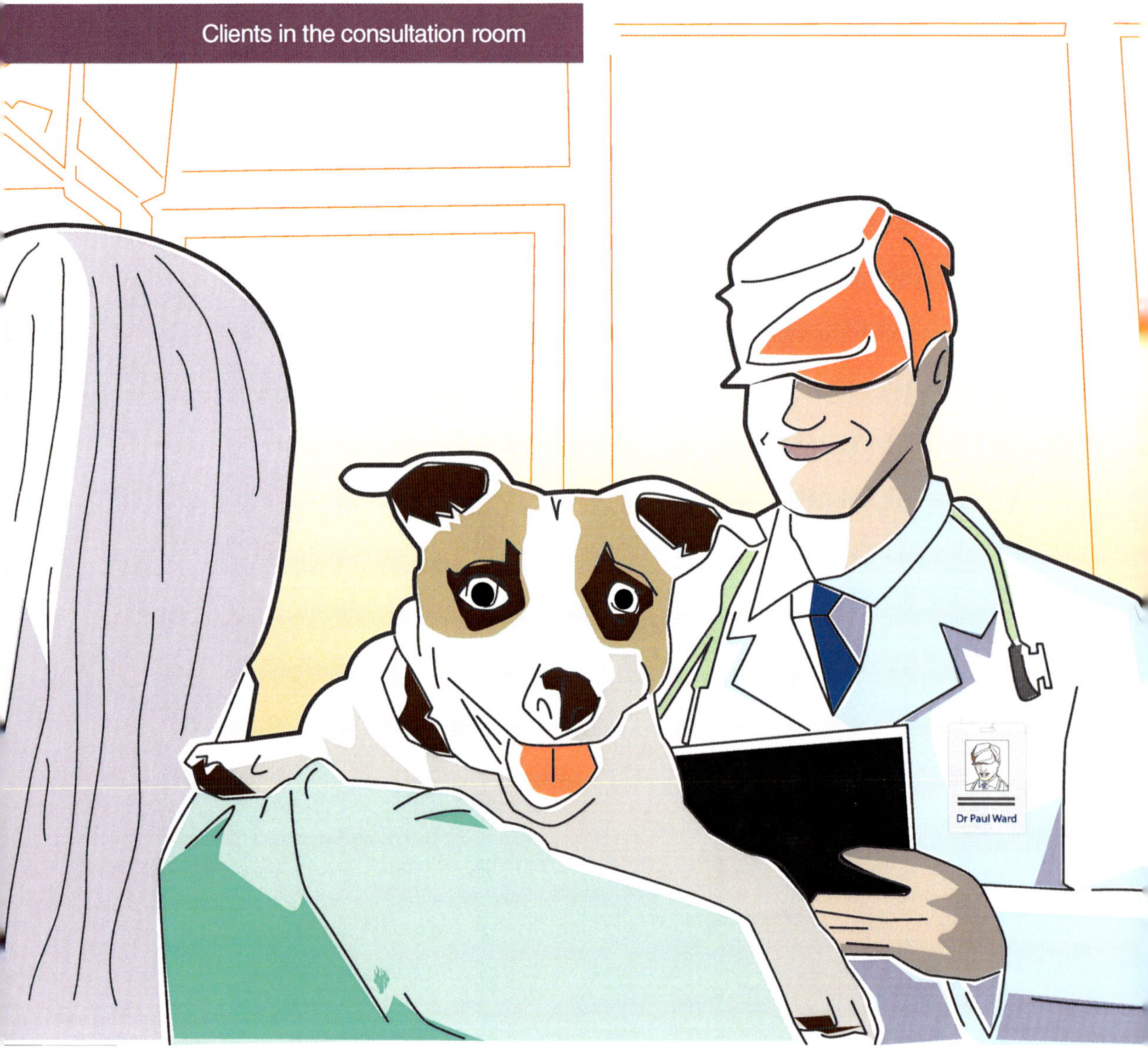

The next stage involves explaining your findings: "Mrs. Campbell, Bobby seems to have diarrhoea. During the physical exam I noticed he is dehydrated, but I would like to run a blood count to confirm this observation. He doesn't have any abdominal pain, so we don't need to take an X-ray for the time being. However, a blood count would provide us with important information about Bobby's health, do you agree that we should collect a blood sample to learn what's wrong?"

You must explain and give reasons. The following points underline some common communication errors:

- Explain what Bobby needs. It is not what you require as a vet, the owner is not interested in your needs. The important thing is what Bobby needs.
- Avoid the use of technical words if you need to explain a blood count. Technicalities will only confuse the owner if they are nervous. Talk in simple terms: "I would like to check whether Bobby has anaemia and his level of white blood cells."
- If you are going to use medical terminology, it is useful to know whether the client is a health professional, so you can omit obvious points and offer a more technical description. Nobody likes to feel foolish, and an error when explaining a blood count to a specialist in internal medicine could make you feel bad and create uncertainty.
- You may perform certain tests and to your surprise the results are normal. This could make you feel guilty for spending the owner's money without obtaining anything conclusive. If this happens, you can approach the owner with the happy news that Bobby is all right and you expect him to get better with the treatment. Highlight that you have ruled out the presence of several significant diseases.
- Also let the client know when you decide tests are unnecessary. This is an important point because it creates future trust. Say things like "I don't think Bobby needs an X-ray today. With the blood count and clinical signs observed during the physical exam, I think we should..." It is vital that you verbalise what the patient does not need, because in the future, when he does need these measures you can say: "You know I would tell you if this test were unnecessary, but Bobby needs it at the moment."

You must check the client has understood everything when prescribing treatments. To stimulate your client's active listening, consider the following points, which are listed according to the order of importance: body language, sounds, spoken language, and written language. It is important to know that only 20 % of what you say stays in the listener's mind, so you must rely on other actions to compensate for this point:

- Look at the client's face and nod your head while speaking.
- Stroking the animal at the same time as the owner will strengthen your connection with the client.
- Speaking (around 20 %) more slowly than normal makes the listener pay more attention.
- Using a softer tone of voice will also receive more attention.
- Repeating points three times throughout the consultation means clients will retain more information.
- Use different means of communication; if you incorporate visual communication along with what you are saying, or take advantage of supporting materials such as written aids or other tangible elements, it will help establish more information in the recipient's mind.
- Ask clients to repeat back how they should administer the treatment to check they have understood the instructions correctly.

Examples of the client's body language

- Some clients do not let go of their animal, using them as defensive barriers to hide behind. They are fearful and do not give their opinion. In such cases, you must withdraw, give them space, and politely ask them to set their pet down on the floor. You must entice them to speak and ask them what is on their mind.
- Younger people usually have a quicker communication style and tend to prefer brisker consultations.
- Older clients require longer visits.
- If the client is in a hurry and constantly looking at their watch, it is better to give them another appointment or ask them if they wish to leave the animal and collect it later. Such a client is not going to listen or pay attention and will not appreciate your work under these circumstances.
- If the owner looks and turns their body towards the door while you are talking, it is because they are rejecting what you are offering them. You must try to change their posture to a more collaborative angle.
- When open to collaboration, the client and vet face each other, for example looking at a document; this is how clients are more likely to accept your proposals.

Designing the consultation room to facilitate communication

Designing spaces is complicated because they are normally created from a perspective that considers ergonomic factors and the operator's workspace. Consultation rooms are designed so you can work efficiently and comfortably, but they often neglect the owner's feelings and how they are affected by their position in the room and its design.

Depending on how long the vet needs to spend examining the patient, the owner may need to sit down. If your consultations are usually quite long, because of a strategic decision to place value on the time you dedicate to each animal, you should consider including seats. However, they are not recommended if you plan for short visits.

Having said this, when handing out an estimate for surgery and support materials, clients are more likely to make a decision when seated. Yet sometimes there is simply not enough room for seats. Therefore, if the client will be standing, you should consider the following points:

- Do not place any clocks where the client can see them.
- Position the client with their back to the waiting room door.
- Design the space so you are on the client's right-hand side, ideally at an angle of 90°, because the client will accept more of your suggestions in this position. If you have to stand up, you can rest any documents or estimates on the examination table.
- Do not place any barriers between you and the client.
- Position computer screens so you do not have to turn your back on the client or turn your body to speak with them. If you turn your back on the client, their brain will subconsciously interpret that you are ignoring them or are unconcerned about what they are saying.
- It is better to avoid playing music in examination rooms because some people are extremely auditory, and their brain will pay more attention to the music than you.

POINTS TO REMEMBER

- Speaking to the client's right ear increases sales by 30 %.
- Gown, logo, and a stethoscope around the neck increase the chances of success by 60 %.
- Around 40 % of people are visual clients.
- Some 20 % are auditory clients.
- The remaining 40 % of people are kinaesthetic, within whom the sense of touch predominates. Knowing how to detect them is a competitive advantage.
- Most clients cannot grade your level of veterinary quality. However, they can measure the quality of your service.
- Speaking 20 % more slowly helps people listen more carefully.
- Speaking 20 % more quietly also increases the effectiveness of your messages.
- As people get older they need more time to think and discuss things, and you should articulate better because they may have poorer hearing.
- Touching the pet while the owner is touching them creates a stronger bond between all of you.

11 Enabling decisions

The everyday activities of a veterinary clinic constantly give rise to situations in which the vet proposes diagnostic tests, treatments, operations, vaccinations, etc., moments when your work is highly dependent on the owner's decision.

Are you prepared to obtain the client's approval? What should you do when the client hesitates?

Strangely enough, clients may occasionally reject your estimate for an operation, and yet they later accept a similar proposal in another practice although there is very little price difference. Can you improve the acceptance level for estimates? Can you learn sales techniques that will enable you to deliver high-quality veterinary medicine?

Veterinary surgeons receive very basic training in sales. Given that we are not tutored in sales at university, we must learn and perfect our sales techniques at a later date.

The vet is often the team member who upholds a price estimate. Larger practices may feature staff trained specifically for this task, but in most clinics, it is something the vet must learn to handle with ease.

Obviously, the final decision about whether to accept an estimate must lie with the owner, thus avoiding future complaints and claims so long as you use an appropriate style of communication and present the options correctly.

You must be familiar with how decision-making processes work, so in this chapter we will discuss biases, the halo effect, claims, statistical presentations, and techniques for presenting more complicated estimates.

Biases

According to the book by Daniel Kahneman, *Thinking, Fast and Slow*, the human mind is continually rewriting stories about the past based on results obtained in the present. Once your mind has a new outlook on things, it rewrites the past to adapt to this new vision. This is called retrospective bias.

For example, if you watch a football match with two evenly matched teams and one of them wins near the end, the mind looks for the strong points of the winning team and makes you believe they were not so equal and you had in fact noticed signs that they were going to win. Further examples are when someone says they knew an economic downturn was coming or a certain disaster was imminent.

Retrospective bias occurs frequently in medicine. One such case is when a complication arises in a low-risk surgical intervention and the patient dies unexpectedly. In hindsight, a panel of experts may be inclined to think the operation involved an unacceptable level of risk or the surgical team failed to execute the technique correctly. This bias rules out the possibility of a neutral retrospective evaluation of a decision that was reasonable when it was made.

Outcome bias is another one you need to know about. It measures skills in function of the results obtained. If an operation has a poor outcome, the owner will think the vet is a bad practitioner; however, if surgery is unexpectedly successful, the veterinary surgeon will be a true hero. The outcome is measured by the story and retrospective evaluation of our work, exaggerating the bias and tipping the scales to one side or the other.

Actions that originally appear cautious, in hindsight may seem irresponsible.

In human medicine, and considering the ever-increasing tendency for legal claims based on negligence, these biases and their consequences have resulted in more diagnostic tests or cases referred to specialists, since the primary care physician wants to avoid unnecessary risks. This can be considered defensive medicine and it is starting to occur in veterinary medicine.

These biases have two possible consequences: either they force the vet to become more cautious, thus avoiding errors; or, if the professional assumes more risk and it turns out all right, they will reinforce their bold approach due to the halo effect.

The halo effect

The halo effect causes people to consider real success stories as if they were heroic victories; for example, the company that started in a garage and is now a multinational corporation, or the professional who developed an empire from nothing and now devotes their fortune to social and humanitarian projects. This effect has a significant impact because it produces admiration and exaggeration in the client, besides adding to your reputation.

The halo effect is also reinforced by an authority bias.

Going back to the Milgram experiment concerning authority (Chapter 10), vets are seen as experts and the authority within their field. If you pressurise the client's decision, using mechanisms such as fear or aggressive sales techniques, the owner will hold you responsible for any treatment failures or unexpected developments in the case, because of the same reasoning derived from the principle of authority.

Claims

Therefore, and to reduce the number of claims, we advise against using the principle of authority to sell veterinary services, even though clients must fill in forms that exclude you from any liability. Word-of-mouth and websites for listing complaints can destroy the reputation of a business.

In human medicine, there is a dramatic reduction in claims when patients and their relatives understand the medical team has done everything within their power to help the patient. This is one of the reasons why you must develop empathy with your patients and their owners and put this commitment into words.

It is very important that you understand these biases, so you can use them appropriately and therefore reduce the number of complaints and help clients reach a decision or make a judgement. You must understand that these are subconscious mechanisms and your ability to influence the owner, one way or the other, depends on your communication technique.

Humans dislike risk and loss.

People select what they believe to be the safest option with the least amount of loss. According to game theory, given the choice between a game in which we can win 90 %, lose 10 %, or take a guaranteed 85 %, we would probably select the last option. However, when given a 50 % chance of winning, we would probably still choose to play.

Yet the percentage of risk is not the only thing that matters; how the professional presents the information can also produce a bias. Here are some examples:

- Surgery always involves some risk. Never use phrases such as "Laboratory tests are not necessary, it is just a routine procedure", "Nothing bad will happen", or "It is insignificant." It is better to use phrases such as "Hopefully everything will turn out all right", "I recommend some routine laboratory tests", etc. The owner must decide, under their own responsibility and after completing an informed consent form, whether or not they want to carry out certain tests.
- You must inform the client of the expected results, underlining the importance of your clinical actions. Even cleaning a patient's mouth can lead to problems due to stress, so you should not understate the clinical procedure or tip the scales towards a fearful situation.
- If you force and abuse the principle of authority, as the vet, you will assume responsibility for what happens, and that is how the client will usually judge the circumstances.

Presenting statistics

Numerous experiments have investigated decision-making in terms of numerical and statistical patterns.

When someone has to undergo a course of chemotherapy and the outlook states that 20 % of patients will be cured while the rest may not overcome their cancer, they are very likely to accept the treatment. However, if they are told chemotherapy is not effective in 80 % of patients, then it is unlikely the patient will agree to undergo the protocol. The statistics are correct in both statements, but how the information is presented has a crucial effect on whether the treatment is accepted. Similarly, we can present the chances of success. Using positive expressions such as "Statistics tell us that 20 % of patients enjoy a better quality of life" can tip the balance in favour of submitting to a treatment.

Let us take another example regarding decision-making. In theory, the choice between several options should make it easier to purchase an item. One supermarket possessed a range of 20 types of shampoo, while another only offered 3 different options, guess which supermarket sold more shampoo? Indeed, it has been demonstrated that sales decrease when more than 7 options are available, and in the present example, 20 possibilities generated more doubts and complicated the consumer's choice. The shoppers touched the products, but the range created confusion in their brains, in fact they were saturated and unable to choose between them. On the other hand, the supermarket with just three brands sold a lot more units.

Transferring this example to the veterinary sector, we can conclude that you should not offer your clients too many options.

More than three medical alternatives will block the reptilian brain, rendering it unable to choose.

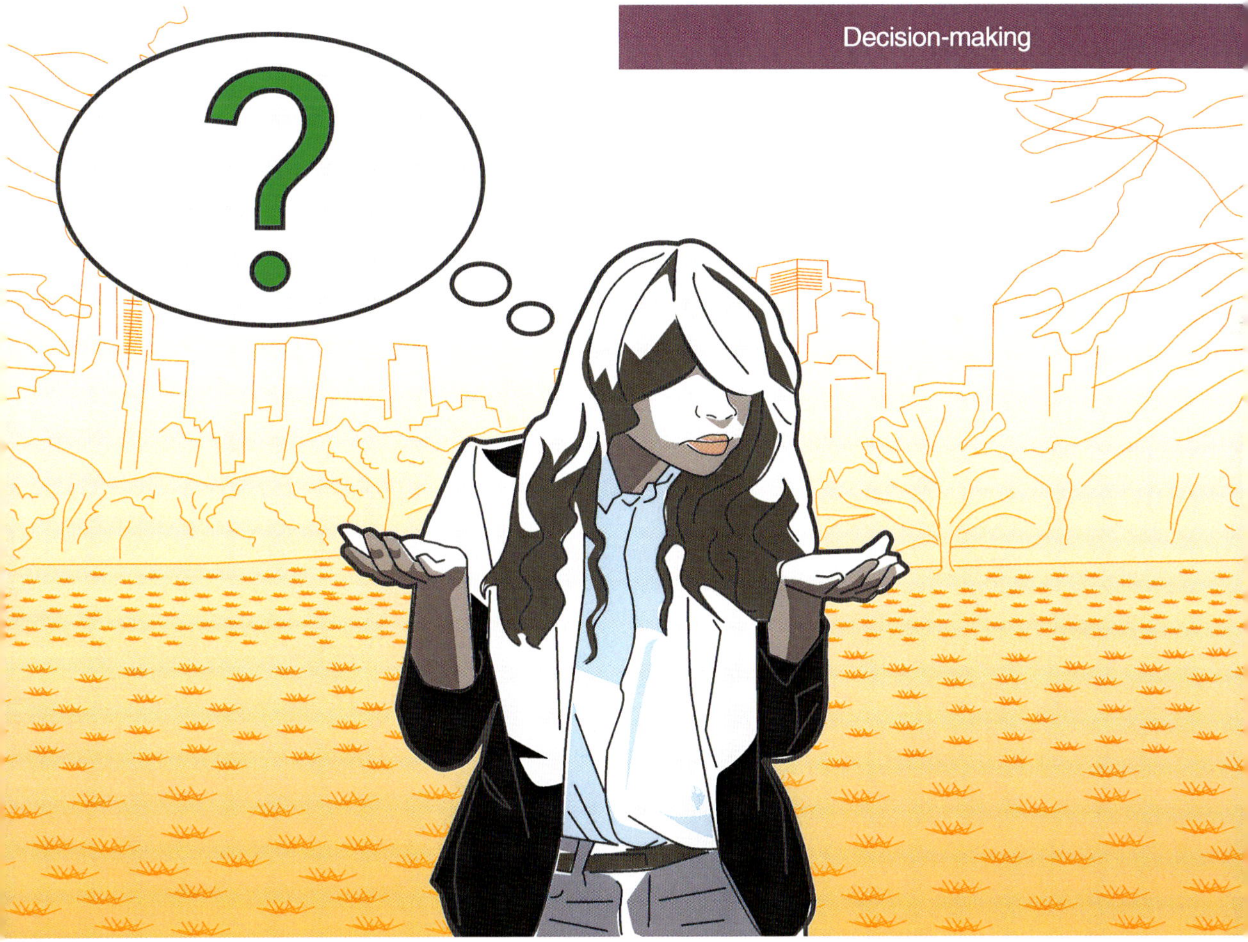

When faced with a complex clinical situation, you must sometimes submit the patient to a lot of tests (biochemical analyses, X-rays, or ultrasound scans) to reach a diagnosis, and the client may find it hard to agree with all these tests at once, even though their animal requires them.

What tools can you use to gain the client's acceptance?

Techniques for presenting estimates

There are two basic techniques for presenting estimates: anchoring and staggering.

Anchoring

This refers to a cognitive bias in which the brain takes a reference point, then uses it as a basis for a decision. Apparently, the mechanism derives from the fact that the brain is unable to differentiate between relevant and irrelevant information.

Cars are often sold using the anchoring technique. Even though the consumer may have seen a television advert, which triggers the decision to buy a car, they enter the dealership with an approximate idea of the car's price. If the salesperson confirms the customer's interest in the car, they will offer a series of discounts. Almost all sales end up with a discussion about the price, which leads the customer to believe they have got a bargain.

Anchoring technique: the salesperson offers a starting price and later reduces it, making the customer feel intelligent, that they know how to negotiate, or are very lucky.

Another example of anchoring is apparent when purchasing materials for your clinic. A sales representative may tell you that a blood chemistry analyser costs €10,000, then say something like "but just this once", "because it is you", "don't tell anybody", or any number of similar phrases, before offering you a 40 % discount, for example. But if you ring a colleague they will probably confirm they received the same offer. A more sophisticated version may require "approval" from an area sales manager or sales executive to close the deal.

The anchor is created by giving the brain a reference. A numeric value is set, then this reference price is used to offer a reduction. If you are initially offered something at a price of €18,000 and eventually buy it for €9,000, you think you have earned a bargain. However, if the starting and final prices are both €9,000, the expenditure will seem fairly high.

How and when should I use anchoring techniques during consultations?

Anchoring is advisable in cases featuring various surgical alternatives, such as a femoral neck fracture in a small dog, where you could offer reconstruction or a femoral head osteotomy. Another example is that of stifle surgery which presents the option of following a classic technique or a more novel technique such as TPLO.

We recommend you start by offering the most advanced technique, with a cost of €XXX, and explain what Bobby needs and that this is the best technique currently available. Ideally the client will accept this option, but they may often ask for discounts or alternatives. You can now offer a different technique and explain that considering Bobby's size and condition you believe it will probably turn out all right and the technique, while rather standard, has at least been tried and tested; furthermore, it costs roughly half the price of the first option. Using the first estimate as an anchor will make the second option seem more acceptable. This is much better than presenting them the other way around.

We advise against dropping your prices or offering discounts on surgical procedures because it devalues your professional prestige and can create mistrust.

If you have given an estimate of €XXX, how can you possibly agree to reduce it later? This produces an unprofessional image, whereas offering an alternative service at a different price can persuade the client to accept one of the two estimates, while you maintain your reputation as a serious professional.

Staggering

This technique is recommended when you need to carry out several tests in a complex clinical case.

Occasionally, some diseases call for a lot of tests to reach a diagnosis. However, it is also known that if you present them all together, the pet owner will probably reject them and request a symptomatic treatment. If the client declines the tests you suggest and the animal gets better following symptomatic treatment, they will be left with the impression that you wanted to make them spend money unnecessarily, thus damaging your future credibility.

Therefore, it is better if you present a rolling estimate, but always based on the patient's clinical picture. You may say something like "Bobby seems to be suffering abdominal pain and vomiting. We should take an X-ray to confirm he hasn't swallowed a foreign object. If the X-ray rules this out, we can proceed with treatment, but if Bobby gets any worse, we may need to perform some further tests."

The advantage of this strategy is that if Bobby gets better, everything is all right and it will generate confidence, but if he gets worse, it is the client who must decide whether to go ahead with the additional tests. The cost will be the same, but it does not produce the same sense of loss because it is carried out in two stages.

Therefore, for each type of service and client, you must know how to handle the situation when giving an estimate or selling a service or product. These techniques must be learnt, the brain will gradually assimilate them to such an extent that staggering an estimate will become just another procedure at the clinic, in the same way you sell a health plan or bundled services.

Knowledge and management of these techniques will also prove useful when dealing with suppliers, as you can recognise and learn to make better purchasing decisions without getting carried away by your impulses.

Other sales techniques

Bundled services

Consumers find it very hard to make a comparison between packages comprising different services. The human mind can compare similar things, but it is much harder to compare combinations.

Bundled packages can be used to sell groups of products (e.g. feed, food bowl, and shampoo in a single set) or veterinary services.

Combinations of medical products are feasible if, for example, they offer checkups for senior patients which include a range of tests, or dental checkups where professional cleaning is combined with a pack for home dental care.

ADVANTAGES OF BUNDLED SERVICES

Increase the client's perception of quality and engagement with their pet.

They are harder to compare between different clinics.

The owner knows the final cost of the complete bundle without having to worry about surprises.

Bundled services are well suited to veterinary surgical procedures. Some examples are:

- The quote for an operation includes four checkups over the next month to monitor the patient's progress.
- Along with the surgery, the price could include two weeks of physiotherapy or acupuncture sessions.
- The price of surgery includes the preoperative laboratory tests and two follow-up X-rays.

Comparisons

This technique is very popular with laboratory sales reps. They offer a product and say that one of your competitors, normally a nearby clinic, has already bought it. The technique activates your sense of competition, as well as your ego, because it provokes a fear of being outdated or losing clients to other veterinary practices, thereby impelling you to make a purchase. It appeals to your sense of need. In terms of your clients, an example would be telling a pet owner that nearly all your patients undergo an annual checkup for vector-borne diseases.

Ego

Salespeople use ego to make consumers feel special and as if they belong to an elite group. The technique is also used extensively in the veterinary sector when reps say something like "Since your centre performs a lot more blood tests than an average clinic, you should own the such-and-such machine." Or in the case of a client who buys an exclusive product, you can tell them very few people can offer their pet such a luxury.

Exclusivity

Exclusivity involves offering a given article at a reduced price for a limited period of time, and to a specific client or groups of clients. In the veterinary industry, suppliers frequently offer special discounts on diagnostic equipment following a conference or for trading in older units, in other words, they may offer the option of trading up your ultrasound for a new one. These offers are normally for a limited period and presented as being specific and exclusive to each customer.

Stories

Product presentations are accompanied by a verbal narrative in which you list the advantages of performing a test, comfortably and quickly, or the greater number of services available if the client makes a certain purchase. The brain visualises the images, and the sensation of experiencing the story makes it lean towards buying the service or product.

Playing with numbers and payment methods

How you present numbers and payment methods can have an influence on whether the client perceives a service as more or less expensive.

Neuromarketing has shown that all figures are compared against a generally higher mental reference. For example, a value of 9.99 is compared to 10, which is the closest round number. Yet a higher value, such as 12, could be viewed as cheaper because the brain will compare it with a reference of 15.

Payment methods are different from the client's point of view. The act of paying involves a release and a sense of loss. This feeling is greater when the loss can be made tangible, especially when paying with cash instead of a credit or debit card.

FINAL RECOMMENDATIONS

1. Always offer the best option first, even though it is the most expensive. The client is more likely to accept it rather than if you offer it after the cheaper alternative.
2. Do not offer more than two or three options because clients will find it hard to make a final decision.
3. If faced with a series of diagnostic tests, present them in a logical order and wait for the first ones to be accepted, then explain further tests may be required depending on the initial results.
4. You should be aware of the different sales techniques you can use to offer your clinic's services. Offer each service using the most appropriate technique based on client type. It will also help you recognise when visiting sales reps are using these techniques.

12 How to offer health plans

This chapter reviews the key points regarding the sale of health plans from a neuromarketing perspective, but first we must give a brief explanation of what health plans are exactly.

What is a health plan?

A pet health plan is a set of services that you offer your clients based on a monthly or annual fee. It generally includes a series of services at no additional cost and some discounted services.

It is your most powerful loyalty-building tool because the owner visits your clinic all year long to take advantage of all the services they have already paid for, that is, hence they do not have to look for the best offer in each clinic. Health plans have been available in some countries since the early 90s, but they only gained popularity more than decade later. Nowadays, clients often ask about them when they visit a veterinary practice.

Therefore, we have dedicated a chapter exclusively to neuromarketing techniques for selling plans.

Key selling points

The chapter's title is correct; we "offer" rather than "sell" health plans because one of the fundamental selling points is to avoid pressurising the client, as they must decide which product is right for them.

There are several keys, which we shall analyse one by one, to opening the client's brain and ensuring they entrust you, as a veterinary surgeon, with the health of their pet.

You owe me one

What happens when you give someone something for free? Unwittingly, this person now feels indebted to you. From this point on, they think about how they can return the favour, how they can rebalance the scale and rid themselves of any debt.

This is known as the **principle of reciprocity** – when you give someone something, they feel obliged to give you something in return. Once the client is benefiting from a health plan, they do not have to pay anything each time they visit you for one of their scheduled appointments included in the plan. If you do your job well, when leaving the client often asks if they owe you anything. When you confirm the service is included in the plan, they may often decide to purchase something from the shop to "compensate" for not spending any money.

Who can compete with the offer of free consultations? If your health plans feature free consultations, no matter how cheap your competition may be, they cannot beat your offer. If you interpret this as giving away your time to clients with a plan, the answer is yes, it is true. Nevertheless, it is even truer that pets whose owners have a health plan are statistically much healthier because they receive regular checkups, unlike animals which only visit the clinic when they are ill.

In fact, every routine appointment is an opportunity to detect health problems early on and intervene before they escalate into something worse. Moreover, given that the visit is free of charge, the client is more likely to approve and pay for complementary diagnostic tests which they may otherwise have declined.

We are practically giving them away!

This works with any type of service or product. If an item is only available at a special price for just one week, many people will buy it impulsively because they know it will cost more later.

This is known as the **principle of scarcity** and we have all occasionally taken the bait. The technique is commonly employed by gymnasiums. Gyms tend to offer promotions after the summer and Christmas holidays, periods in which many people consume too much food and drink; for example, no joining fee, one week's free trial, or a free locker when paying a year's full membership. It attracts new members through an explosive combination. They know you want to do something about your excess weight, so they make it easy for you.

The same thing applies to health plans. Pet owners are more inclined to purchase plans when they have more money (e.g. after receiving their annual bonus). Offer plans with a special incentive at this time of year and new clients will acquire them.

The vet told me

Owners enter clinics in search of a veterinary surgeon, in other words, an expert in animal medicine. Do not disappoint them. They are there to find a solution to their pet's health problem, they will find it hard to respect you as a vet if your clothing is dirty or old, if the clinic looks more like a shop than a medical centre, or if it is full of bad odours. All these points would damage your credibility.

The clinic and staff must portray a pristine, professional image.

If you present a pristine appearance, you can take advantage of the **principle of authority**, as explained in the previous chapter. As such, clients will accept your opinion as a veterinary professional regarding the best means of looking after their pet's health, for example, in the form a health plan.

All pets would benefit from a health plan because they include all the checkups, vaccinations, and laboratory tests recommended for each stage of the pet's life, besides the advantage of being able to visit your clinic whenever the need arises.

If the vet says so, then it must be good for my pet.

It is the best option for your pet

We must also discuss the **principle of consistency**. Responsible owners, those who love their pet as if they were another member of the family, are the target audience. If they have no financial limit, they will always try to do the very best for their pet, but as the vet, you are responsible for teaching them how to do it.

In the case of an illness, when you offer them several treatment alternatives or diagnostic tests, the client will often ask you what you would do in their position. Just be honest and tell them: "The best thing for Bobby would be to conduct some blood and urine tests, so we can evaluate his kidney and pancreatic function." This sort of expression is not too bad. In fact, this is what most vets would normally say. However, to make your recommendations more effective, you should start by saying something like "How concerned are you about Bobby's state of health?"

The answer to this question leads you onto the next one, thus giving you the opportunity to offer the most appropriate tests.

If the client tells you they are very worried, and they are coherent with this reply, the owner will probably agree to the tests you recommend as well as any subsequent treatment you deem necessary. However, if they are not too concerned, your sales pitch should steer towards suggesting the same tests, but whilst also offering some alternatives, such as a staggered proposal for tests: "We could start with a urine test to check Bobby's urine concentration, which will help us determine if he has a kidney problem, and his glucose in urine level, which would confirm the presence of a pancreatic problem. If we do not obtain conclusive results, we will have to perform more tests."

This means that even the clients who are less "committed" to their pets will not feel pressurised, whereas the concerned client will be coherent and follow your recommendations.

A large smile

The first three seconds are essential for earning your client's trust through their primitive brain. An honest, open smile that produces laugh lines at the sides of your eyes makes anyone relax, lowers their level of alertness, and subdues potential preconceptions. There is no better cover letter.

Even if you are having a bad day, your last client was overly insistent, or the telephone has not stopped ringing, none of these problems are the fault of your next client, and you must always treat them as someone special.

Questionnaires conducted in veterinary clinics, and any other type of business, all reveal that **friendliness** is held in higher regard than knowledge, ease of parking, or prices. I think you will agree that it is worth the effort.

Sometimes it can be hard to smile when faced with an angry client, but you must force yourself (albeit in a controlled manner) in order to reduce the tension. This point is covered in greater detail in Chapter 15, where we discuss how to deal with complaints.

Nearly all my clients have purchased a health plan for their pet

People are sheep, or lemmings, call them what you will. Either way, humans tend to follow the herd. Most of us do not swim against the tide, and when something becomes fashionable, we usually follow the trend, either consciously or subconsciously. Our brains will justify the decision later if somebody questions our choice.

Television adverts are always making claims such as "9 out of 10 dentists use XXX toothpaste", which combine the principles of authority and social coherence, thus converting it into a much more powerful message. Another example is when a detergent manufacturer states that all the top dishwasher brands recommend their product.

Accordingly, you can make use of the **principle of social coherence**. When you have been offering plans for quite a while, you could use an expression like "Nearly all my clients have purchased a health plan." Or a better opening phrase might be: "Since we've been offering health plans, almost all of our clients have signed up for one."

Faced with this information, the client feels compelled to buy one, they do not want to be the exception. It is not a question of lying, but rather convincing the owner to purchase a plan and ensure the best care for their pet.

Develop your sales pitch

Now you have all the tools and it is time to put the theory into practice, to create your message or slogan that embeds your clinic in the consumer's mind.

Of course, you must prepare a sales pitch in your own words, a story that incorporates all the elements mentioned previously, and then recount it with sincerity. You need to formulate a straightforward and an elaborate version of your story to fit each situation.

The longer version is easier to write but boring your audience would be ill-advised. Explaining your main strength and three most powerful messages should suffice. The objective is for your future client to enter into a conversation in which they can raise any issues they would like to ask you about.

Recommendation: start with the shorter version, which is known as the elevator pitch.

Your sales pitch

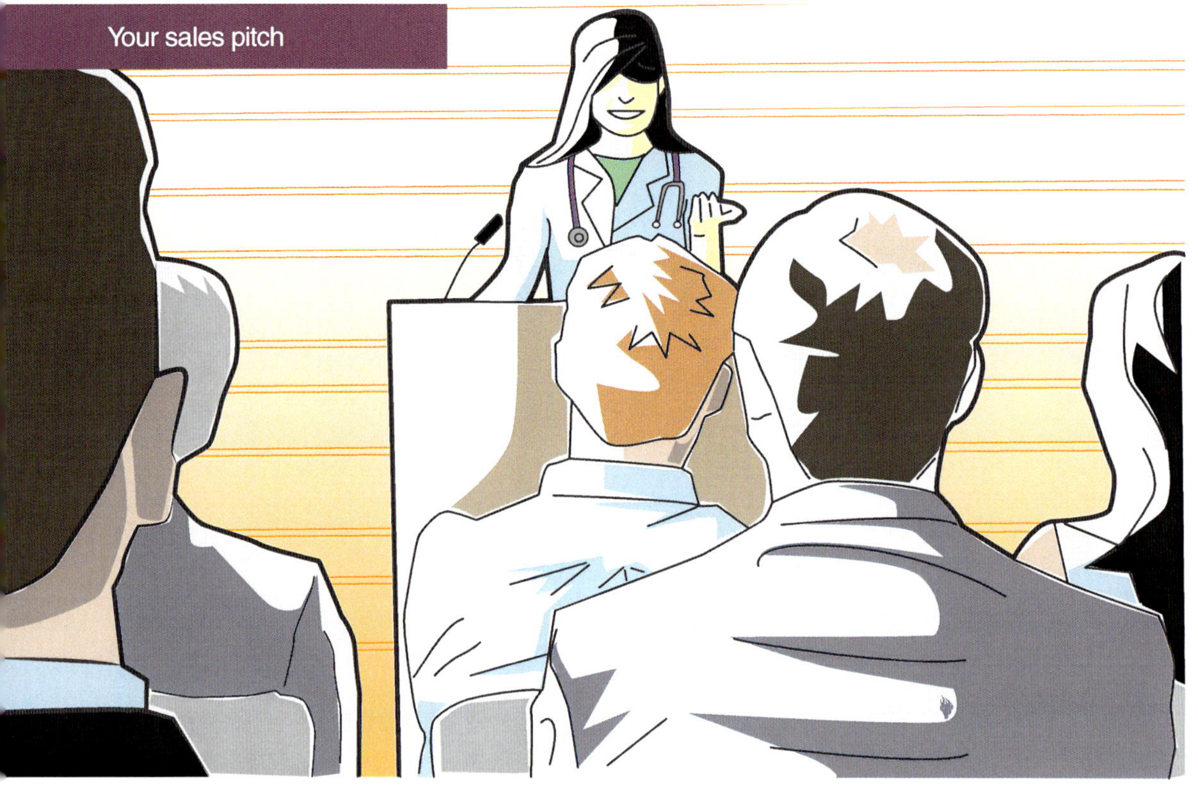

Summarising your message in less than a minute is no mean feat, but as a reward you will be able to sell your services to anyone, even if they have very little time available. This 30–60 second period (although some people allow up to 2 minutes) is the time you may spend with someone in an elevator, for example, or with other businesspeople during a networking session, or with clients during a social event held at your clinic.

Your pitch will be more striking and easy to remember if you can transmit your message in just a few words. What is more, it will give interested listeners time to ask about specific points which you can then explain in more detail.

With time, you will gradually perfect your story. Seize every opportunity to present your pitch in public as you will become increasingly persuasive with practice.

Given the popularity of Twitter, there is a tendency to simplify messages even further, boiling them down to less than 140 characters, or roughly 20 words. Condensing everything into one sentence is a challenge. Are you up for it?

13 Even more complicated: neuromarketing on social media

"Instant success", which is what every veterinary surgeon seeks for their clinic, is an oxymoron. Success is always the product of a long process, nevertheless, the use of social media (SM) can accelerate this process. Therefore, we shall now discuss how to develop a neuromarketing strategy for the internet, since most SM will have disappeared within 10 years after reading this book. Sales strategies for products and services will, however, still be valid and adapt to the new channels.

New clients will not only reach your clinic through the front door or by telephone, but also by means of SM and your company website. Starting with a well-designed website, you should structure your presence in other social media, so your messages are coherent and to avoid duplicating content, for example, by repeating blog content on your website.

Neuromarketing has shown that we have to conquer the consumer's mind with eye-catching images. They are much more effective than text. Employ images of animals, people hugging animals – appeal to the client's protective and neotenic instincts (the puppy principle). Companies are already developing odour printers: soon you will be able to smell the websites you visit; can you imagine how that will revolutionise the sale of perfumes?

The human mind is designed to follow movement, that is why designers have developed banners and moving images that appear in website headers. Another basic principle of advertising to bear in mind, which has been measured and tested in neuromarketing studies, is that humans turn their attention to what the person in front of them is looking at.

EXAMPLE

If you are running a campaign through your website headers, you can position a dog beneath them looking towards the phrase you want your clients to read.

You must endeavour to be coherent when working with SM. Never portray an image that differs from your reality because it would create mistrust in the client's mind. Using real images of your clinic emanates authenticity and shows you have nothing to hide. If one or two people work at the clinic, make them visible with photographs; on the other hand, if your clients are surrounding veterinary practices, you will have to design a professional-oriented website in addition to the clinic's website. Consequently, the following is very important: you must know who you are and who your client is.

NOTE

This chapter is predominantly practical, so please get a pen and paper and ready yourself for some exercises.

Know who you are

Before considering the target audience, you must know who you are and what you offer. Only then can you identify who your ideal client is, the market niche you want to focus on, and the message you wish to transmit, and subsequently appeal to their specific purchasing criteria. If you skip over some of the steps, you will not obtain the same result.

Personal brand and differential value proposition

The theory is simple; in order for your audience to desire your services, you must define your personal brand and what makes you special. Otherwise, you are just another veterinary clinic. A lot of companies spend most of their time and resources fighting for their market position. Yet rather than spending so much energy competing, why not turn your attention to finding new markets without any competition? This is the focus of the theory of blue and red oceans.

THE THEORY OF BLUE AND RED OCEANS

The traditional red ocean strategy (a cutthroat market stained red with blood) entails competing in an established market (e.g. against normal veterinary clinics), challenging the competition, and adopting different strategies to occupy a place in the market (e.g. cutting costs to lower prices, offering the best service available, etc.). In other words, positioning yourself with respect to others.

The blue ocean strategy avoids competition by focusing on innovation and creating a market in areas that are yet to be exploited. In the veterinary sector, clinics for cats or exotic animals could serve as examples of the most recent red oceans, while the first ones were speciality clinics.

Find your blue ocean and your message will go viral across the internet.

If you are still searching for your blue ocean and competing in bloody waters, at the very least you must identify your differential value proposition (DVP). To this end, you must identify the service you can offer and which nobody else is offering.

EXAMPLE

A pet day care/boarding service where clients can leave their pets while they are on holiday or at work, with the added benefit of giving the vet an opportunity to administer vaccinations or carry out any pending tests or analyses. It would still be a traditional veterinary clinic, but with an innovative service.

If you are going to offer a new service, always emphasise the benefits for the end user and link them to the image of a happy animal – make neuromarketing work for you.

EXERCISE

Write down your DVP.

Define your ideal client

Now you know who you are, you can identify your target audience. It may be self-evident, but if your flagship service is a pet day care centre, your average client is unlikely to be looking for low prices, and vice versa.

You need to put a face on your ideal client, their habits, lifestyle, education, family status, etc. Obviously, not all clients will fall into this stereotype, but if these are the type of clients you want, your messages must be coherent in order to reach them and avoid wasting energy on attracting others.

In the example of the clinic with a pet day care service, the typical client would have the following characteristics: medium/upper class, single, good income, workaholic. Therefore, you would have to find the social media this client visits and advertise there.

EXERCISE

Describe your ideal client in as much detail as possible.

Talk in terms of benefits

Talking about objective facts is not very helpful in the world of neuromarketing. The primitive brain is not interested in these matters. Pleasure and the benefit derived from doing something do, however, capture its attention. Continuing with the example of the day care service, an objective client will react positively to the following message: "While you work, we will look after Toby and ensure he is happy and has a good time." Or in the case of a neutering procedure, to overcome the owner's resistance, it is better to say: "It is preventive surgery, and Bella can soon return to playing with her friends in the park", instead of "Spaying will reduce the chance of Bella developing tumours." Both statements are true, but the first one is positive and presents a benefit, while some people may find the second rather painful.

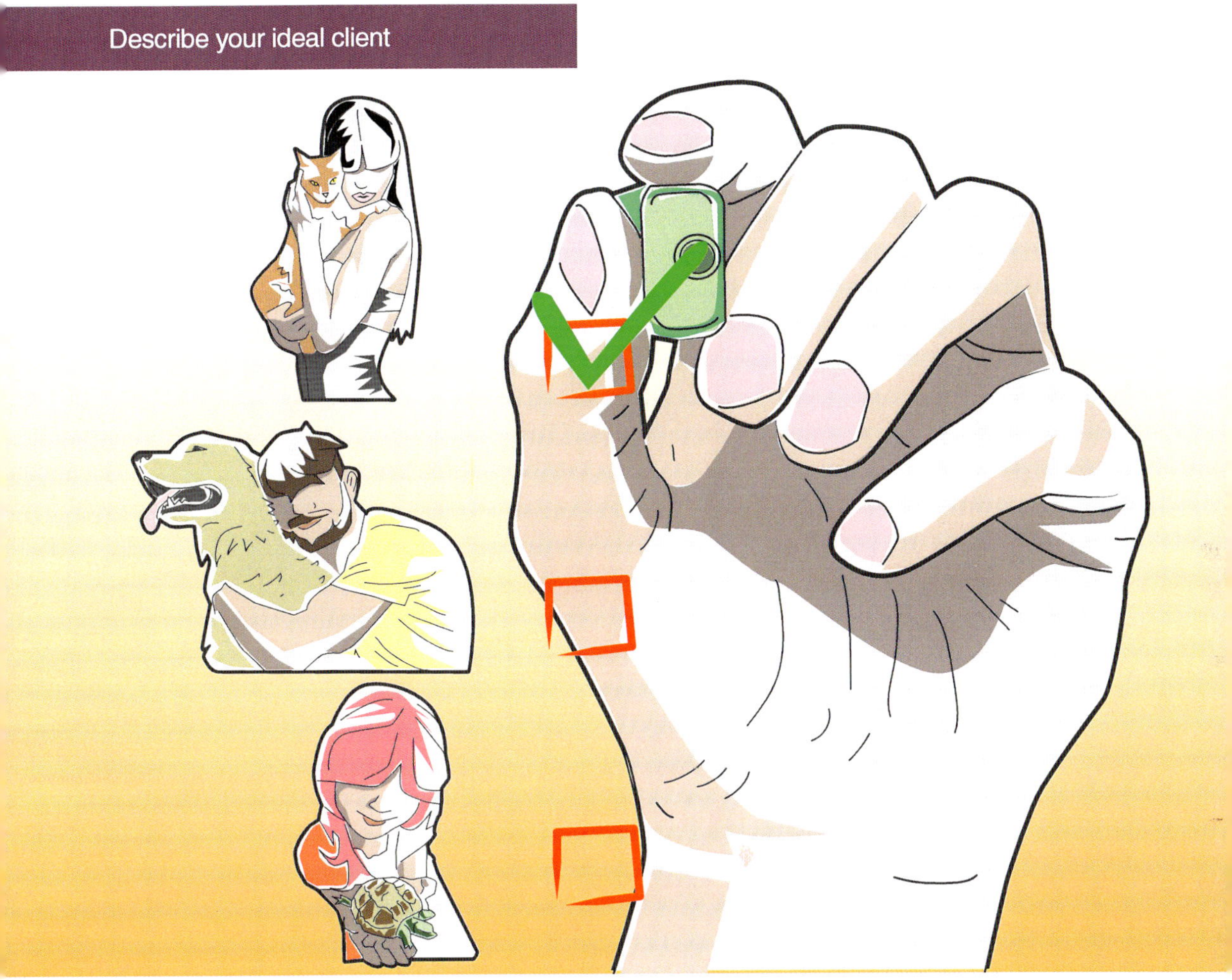

While discussing positive phrases, we should also mention positive and not so positive words. Seed words are those which arouse positive ideas. Joy, affection, birth, growth, future, investment, wellbeing, opportunity, new, synergy, etc., all sound better than negative words such as cancer, disease, problem, no (this is the worst, always try to avoid it), expensive, difficult, etc. Ensure that you only express yourself with the first group when talking to the client.

EXERCISE

Use seed words to write a phrase that reflects the benefits offered by your clinic.

Purchasing incentives

We are all motivated by different interests. We each have a switch that awakens our interest to purchase a product or service. The four basic stimuli we seek in a service or when purchasing a product are: innovation, price, affection or pleasure, and safety or comfort.

Going back to the pet day care service, in this case the ideal client is essentially looking for convenience, as the price does not represent a problem for them, whereas clients at low-cost clinics are in pursuit of a cheap vaccination.

Neuromarketing plan

Once you have identified your target audience and DVP, you are ready to draw up your marketing plan. In the present case it will be a neuromarketing plan because your budget is probably smaller, and you must address the basic needs of your future clients.

First decide who will undertake this task. Can you imagine who it will be?

The clinic's community manager

That's right, you will take on this job. Or at least you must be kept in the loop.

A veterinary clinic is no different from any other business and, as such, you could employ a professional community manager to handle your SM marketing. Above all, however, we are veterinary surgeons who work with patients and clients, and it is hard for someone outside the clinic to create your messages. A community manager without a veterinary background cannot write a post about something as straightforward as preventing leishmaniasis or advice on how to maintain pet's skin health, let alone a clinical case you wish to publish. Nevertheless, they would be able to help disseminate your message and find the most appropriate channels for publishing each type of information.

In the case of large clinics, it is worth assigning part-time SM management duties to one of the auxiliary staff or vets, so your message is disseminated from within the clinic, or you could hire a community manager, possibly a client. If they are unfamiliar with your clinic, they will not provide a true reflection of your business and your message will not get through.

As regards small clinics, you will probably have to take charge of creating and publishing the content. Focus your attention on just one social network and get organised. We will explain how to do this later.

EXERCISE

Write the name of the people who will take charge of SM in your clinic and describe their functions. At least two people should be involved.

Search engine optimisation (Google SEO and SEM)

Gaining visibility on the internet costs time (Search Engine Optimisation, SEO), money (Search Engine Marketing, SEM), or both. Ideally you should invest a bit of time and some money, as it is hard for most vets to free up enough time to write content on a regular basis. Search engines used to place more weight on the publication of original content, but nowadays you have to pay to appear on Google's first page. In fact, 60 % of browsers select one of the first three search results on the list.

TIP

Post new content as often as possible (weekly, fortnightly, or monthly) and pay to place advertisements as well.

EXERCISE

Set aside 1 % of your annual turnover to invest in SM. Divide this amount by 12 to calculate your monthly advertising expenditure.

Content curation

We will discuss what to publish or where to publish it later, but first you must determine the content you wish to share to obtain engagement (interaction between the consumer and your brand). Content curation is the ability to find, filter, and make use of information gleaned from a range of different sources, before finally adding a personal touch and then presenting it for your audience's interest.

It is as straightforward as requesting notifications from Google Alerts each time something new is published in one of your favourite areas, so you can share and reflect on these reports; or learning about current topics and offering your opinion on them, with the aid of Google Trends. Both applications are easy-to-use and free, but many others are available.

> **EXERCISE**
> Enter your Gmail account and sign up for Google Alerts and Google Trends. Read what is written about your topics of interest and share it. Get inspired and write about it.

Planning content. Editorial calendar

Do not think the job is done just because you know who you are, your target audience, and what you are going to present, but this is the first step and it will give your message coherence. The first objective is to occupy a place in the client's mind, the second is to refresh this presence with a suitable frequency.

New tools will emerge, but we shall now explain two tools that are free and easy-to-use (Google Calendar and Hootsuite).

Create an editorial calendar by selecting the topics you are going to cover over the next 12 months (or 52 weeks, depending on your availability and that of your team) and record them in the agenda or an Excel sheet. Next, choose the media through which you will publish your content and finally schedule the publications.

If December's theme is leishmaniasis, you should create or share news items about this topic and publish them on Facebook, for example. After organising the month's articles and news, you can set a reminder in Google Calendar to publish on the given date or use Hootsuite to schedule the publication in advance. We recommend you dedicate one morning or afternoon each month to writing and selecting the content, then set up a schedule to publish it through Hootsuite. As such, you won't have to do anything else until the following month. Rainy days are perfect for writing content.

> **EXERCISE**
> You know what you have to do, write your editorial calendar. Select this year's 12 topics of interest and create a Hootsuite account to schedule their publication.

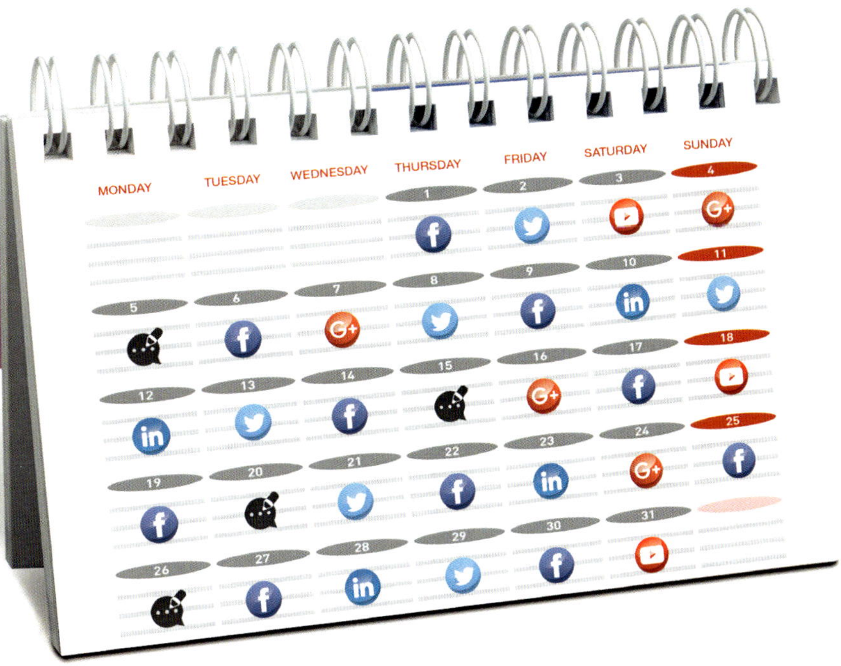

Example of an editorial calendar

Segment clients

Specific content is suitable for specific clients. There is no sense in sending cat owners information about leishmaniasis for a month, nor should you send content on reptile hibernation to clients with dogs. They might be interested in it, but it is better to segment your database and direct your messages more effectively.

We suggest you maintain all your clients' email addresses up-to-date (with their prior written permission to respect data protections laws) and create different client lists, so you can offer them services that fit in with their needs. Besides general lists organised according to species (dogs, cats, birds, ferrets, rabbits, etc.), you can create groups of elderly pets, those with kidney disease, dermatological problems, puppies, to name but a few examples. Each list of clients will receive content that is better adapted to their needs.

EXERCISE

Create your species-specific emailing lists. You will create some more later, but do not fret, we shall take it step by step.

Capture subscribers

Your first goal was to obtain these emails and generate emailing lists with segmented clients. Now your objective is to convince these clients to follow your publications. This can be achieved by different means: asking them to click on the "like" button in Facebook or your blog, or by using email marketing.

Email marketing is the mass sending of emails to a group of contacts (which is why it is important to segment your clients into lists), so your message will reach them all directly by means of just a single action. There are several tools available, but the easiest to use are MailChimp and Mailrelay, which are also free. Alternatively, you can make client lists in your habitual email server and send out the emails by more traditional methods.

EXERCISE

If you have time, open a MailChimp or Mailrelay account and learn how they work by watching some internet tutorials.

The aim is to build loyalty

SM channels are not ideal for sales, you should use them to present your services to future clients and help retain existing ones. Regard SM as a tool based around the generosity of users, which provides valuable information for pet owners, as a credible reference, and a trustworthy channel.

You want to transmit the following message: "The free content I'm receiving from this clinic is so good, then the services they provide at the centre must be excellent."

Some experts say you should publish content following the four-to-one ratio, in other words, for every four interesting, informative, or entertaining publications, present one publication that contains a commercial offer or proposal. Ideally, only offer promotions from time to time. The only exception to this rule is the case of low-cost clinics, as they seek a high number of clients as opposed to high-quality clients.

EXERCISE

Write down 12 commercial messages linked to each of the monthly topics.

Everything begins with your website and Google Maps: why my clinic?

This is the question you must ask yourself: why does your clinic exist? As mentioned earlier, you don't exist unless you have internet presence. It may be cruel, but it is the simple truth. You must have a website and feature on Google Maps. This comes before publishing anything in SM. Luckily, you already know what you are selling (assuming you have read and implemented the preceding chapters). The following are some key points to ensure your clients find you easily and like what they see.

EXERCISE

Check your website can be viewed correctly on all devices and your clinic appears on Google Maps. If not, make the necessary changes.

The rule of three

Browsers will not be very interested in what you have to say if your content includes too much information or text. Your website's home page should offer three ideas, three concepts, and three clear images. Less is more.

It is better to incorporate three large, attractive photos, with just one clear message or title, and an invitation to read more by clicking on a link, rather than paragraphs of beautifully written text which nobody will read. The idea is to seduce your browsers.

EXERCISE

Write down the three main ideas you want to convey through your website and confirm it reflects these messages. If it doesn't, make the necessary changes.

Social approval

You must familiarise yourself with the principles of influence in order to seduce your clients. There are many, but perhaps the most powerful is the principle of social approval; being aware that other people visit your clinic. That is why setting aside one of the three main windows on your website for publishing client testimonials could be an excellent idea. They could be written comments, accompanied by a photo of the client with their pet, but a video is even better.

EXERCISE

Ask your best clients to write a testimonial and publish it on your website and/or favourite social media.

Principle of scarcity

The principle of scarcity is another very effective means of influencing the consumer's mind.

If you advertise a 4-month-long neutering campaign, for example, the client's mind will interpret the following message: "I've got plenty of time, I'll do it next month."

However, if you say "only available to the first 10 clients", or "this offer ends in 7 days", the call or necessity effect transforms it into a more powerful sales mechanism. A campaign should include definitive start and end dates and must never be extended.

Considering this time element, it is better to publish special offers on landing pages instead of directly on your website. Additionally, this will provide information about the client's origin and the marketing impact of the current offer.

You can also offer the chance to print discount coupons to help promote services or campaigns. The words "free" and "discount" attract a lot of attention from consumers and encourage them to return to your website regularly in search of new offers.

EXERCISE

Write a campaign based around the principle of scarcity.

Reinvent yourself or die

If your website is more than 5 years old, then it is time to update or completely redesign it. Maybe it doesn't load correctly on smartphones or tablets, which are now used to look up information with a much higher frequency than PCs and laptops. Just as we all have to upgrade our computer equipment, websites must also modernise and adapt to the times and changes in coding. In 2018, designing websites with WordPress is still relevant, but by 2025 new platforms will be available or the present ones will have evolved. Check whether your logo is old-fashioned or needs reworking.

EXERCISE

Ask your friends what they think about your website, whether it appears modern or old-fashioned. Now that you have identified the messages you want to get across, hire a webmaster to renew your website in WordPress.

Reviews in Google and Facebook

Reviews on Google (Google My Business) and Facebook ratings are just as effective as testimonials published on your website, if not more so. We all look at them before selecting a restaurant, hotel, or health resort. Potential clients do the same thing with veterinary practices.

A video is worth a thousand pictures

Some idioms have become outdated: "A picture is worth a thousand words."

In the digital age, things develop at the speed of light. As mentioned earlier, media channels will change, but images and especially videos will always have a greater impact on the consumer's mind than a very well written article or a long list of characteristics, no matter how interesting they may seem.

Storytelling

Alright, so you are going to record a video, but you must write the script first. There is a magic formula for writing a great script that pulls on the audience's heartstrings – tell a story. Storytelling involves narrating a fact-based tale that emotionally touches the viewer. What is more, if it is your own personal story, it will have an even greater impact.

EXERCISE

Write a powerful, fact-based story. Do not exceed 1 minute. Tell it to others at every opportunity. Once you have memorised it well, record it on video.

YouTube

Once you have recorded the video, the public must be able to see it, you need to make them aware of it. You could publish it on your favourite social network and/or upload it to YouTube. It involves more work, but you will earn more prestige if you have your own YouTube channel and organise your videos in themed playlists. An essential playlist for your YouTube channel is the one that features client testimonials. As such, you should upload the videos on your website to your YouTube channel. Do not forget to label all the videos, this will help direct relevant traffic to your website from search engines.

EXERCISE

Open a YouTube account and create your own channel with several playlists: testimonials, dogs, cats, clinical cases, etc.

Guerrilla marketing

Wikipedia defines guerrilla marketing as "a collection of strategies and techniques implemented using unconventional methods and which achieve their goal through ingenuity and creativity rather than heavy investment in traditional advertising spaces". This form of advertising captures the target audience's attention more effectively thanks to its originality. SM represents a quick, free route to guerrilla marketing.

Smartphones are your best friend

If you want to avoid the complication of using a digital camera to make an attractive and original video or photo, a smartphone always makes an excellent resource for effortless guerrilla marketing. Everyone carries a smartphone in their pocket, and I assure you there is nothing more successful on a social network than a photo of a pet being hugged by their owner. It easily beats a beautifully written article or the invention of the century, plus it is very handy.

With the tools available today, it is as easy as taking a photo with your mobile, retouching it on the go with some photo-editing software (you can use Instagram and post it there at the same time) and uploading it to Facebook, Twitter or your favourite social media. Get your entire team involved in this task and you will be sure to succeed.

Speaking of smartphones, there are mobile apps that link the client directly to your clinic, so they can request an appointment or post an image of their pet. This reinforces the connection and sense of belonging that the reptilian brain loves so much. Furthermore, it reassures clients that you are always there for them. Does anything create a stronger bond than presence and proximity?

EXERCISE

Take a photo with your mobile every day and post it on your social media. With time, you can perfect the habit by retouching photos when necessary.

Designing your advertisements

It is worth investing a few extra minutes to make sure your adverts are as appealing as possible. Using basic, free graphic design software (www.canva.com, for example) you can insert text and diagrams on the photo and work with templates to adjust the format to fit different social networks. In other words, you can use it to design your Facebook cover photo or your Twitter and YouTube profiles.

EXERCISE

Create a Canva account and design your first Facebook cover photo. It is really easy.

Publish your posts regularly

That's right, an attractive cover photo is not enough, you must upload content on a regular basis. An inactive Facebook page, a Twitter account without any tweets for at least 6 months, or an Instragram profile that you abandoned 20 weeks ago all embody dormant social media activity. If you cannot do it yourself, assign the job to one of your team members. Remember it is better to focus on participating actively on just one social network where you reply to users, instead of having three open but unattended social media accounts.

Interaction with the public in the form of likes, sharing, and discussions is very well rewarded in terms of positioning on social media sites. It is worth publishing high-quality content (even if not very often) and sharing news from other sources that adds value to the social network.

TIP

Always remember to use an appropriate tone of language. If you are addressing other veterinary professionals because you own a referral practice, use technical and professional language. However, most practices address the needs of pet owners. Use straightforward language, avoid technical words, respond to clients quickly, and, above all, do not post any unpleasant photographs or which contain blood. Nobody wants to imagine their animal in such a situation.

Each social network has its own language. If you are inexperienced in the matter, create a fictitious profile and practice. On Facebook, for example, over two-thirds of your clients are women, so you should use neoteny, photos of puppies, and the idea of protection. Most of your Facebook followers are your clients, so use it as a loyalty-building tool.

Your website, on the other hand, is your brand image and must be well-positioned. It should include more professional articles, but without going too far. Always bear in mind that your clients are not vets. It is better to use a blog to publish more technical topics.

Use Instagram to post photos of clients with their pets and link them to your website. This will produce a high repost rate as people love to share photos of "their furry babies".

You must monitor your analytics to learn about the efficacy of your work on social media. When measuring content, it is important to remember factors such as time on page; the visitors may well be reading your posts if it is more than 3 minutes. Furthermore, you should measure the average number of visits to your site and how many new users you attract. You can obtain all this information from Google Analytics for Google, in WordPress statistics, and in the statistics for your Facebook page, and it will help you decide what time and date to publish and which content is most successful.

In the same vein, remember to ask your new clients how they learned about your services, whether through Facebook, an advertisement, or a friend's recommendation, so you can discover which is your most effective channel.

EXERCISE

Concentrate on just one social network and spend 5 minutes a day replying to your followers' comments. Write one article per week and share another two or three interesting items using Google Trends and Google Alerts.

Change your cover photo regularly

Changing your social media cover photo/banner is free, and you can do it using Canva. The idea of creating a perpetually attractive cover photo is old-fashioned. Take the opportunity to include your monthly proposal in your Facebook cover photo or adapt your Twitter header with the latest #Hashtag. You could also match your YouTube banner with your Facebook cover photos or make them completely different. For example, they could cover the same topic you scheduled in your calendar but with a different image, or deal with a different concept. The choice is yours.

TIP

Never neglect the quality and content of the photos you post. Remember clients expect to see neoteny, pleasant images, and happy people. Never include unpleasant scenes. We recommend the use of light backgrounds to avoid eyestrain.

EXERCISE

Have you got the time and energy? Design your 12 cover photos for this year and save them in a folder. You will just have to change them at the beginning of each month.

Well-written text is still important

Nevertheless, dear reader, please don't be fooled. Of course, images have become more important than text, but they must be accompanied by a caption or tag that attracts the browser's attention. The words used to describe the content will influence the number of people who open your post, email, or video.

Copywriting

To close the loop, does writing come naturally to you or do you need help? Most publications posted on SM do not require any special skills, but some help is always well-received if you are going to write regularly. You could take a course on copywriting to improve your ability to capture the attention of your target audience, that is, your future clients.

Here are two basic tips:

- Try to keep your texts within a limit of 140 characters (or ideally less than 100), so you can post them on any social media platform without editing. Nobody likes to read more than this.
- Transform your headlines or the start of your messages into a poke in the eye. This is a strong phrase, but it is very descriptive. If the beginning of your message grabs their attention, they will continue reading. Otherwise, they will continue browsing until something interests them.

An extra tip: the use of humour is always helpful, but only when appropriate.

EXERCISE

Get used to writing short text with attention-grabbing headlines. If you can, complete a copywriting course.

Why do I need a blog?

Just as you defined an editorial calendar, you must contemplate the main theme for your blog. You can classify the topics to be covered into as many categories as you wish, but it is better to concentrate on a handful of core ideas to simplify the objective of reaching your target followers. The WordPress platform is free unless you want to own a shorter, more individual domain name (i.e. you have to pay to remove the ".wordpress" part), but it is still good value for money.

Blog entries should be marked in red on your editorial calendar. You should post new material at least once a month, or ideally on a weekly basis. This would require collaboration from your staff, but if this is impractical, once a month will be enough (but every month without fail).

Extra tip: prepare a perk for people who subscribe to your blog and want to access special content, so they will earn a reward after giving you their details. It could be a list of dos and don'ts, a special tip, or a discount. Everyone likes free gifts.

EXERCISE

Open a WordPress account and create your blog. Write about the topics in your editorial calendar.

Guest blogger

The next step, once your blog is up and running, is to try to write in other people's blogs. You need to find and interact with other bloggers who write about the same topics.

How do you go about this? Spend a few weeks writing comments on most of their posts. Once they know who you are (not everyone writes comments), offer to write an article on their blog. Most bloggers would ask to see the text before posting it, so they can check the quality is acceptable. If they like it, they will say yes – they are unlikely to turn down the chance of a week off without having to rack their brains in search of a new topic to write about.

In the worst case scenario the blogger says no, but you haven't lost anything. They will probably ask you to return the favour, and therefore you will get a week off from writing a post.

EXERCISE

Research and read blogs written by other vets to get some ideas and topics to write about. Ask if you can write in their blog and invite them to post something in yours.

Press releases

Writing press releases is more difficult, unless your friend is a journalist. If not, search the internet for journalists who are involved with animals and get in touch with them. They will be interested to hear your newsworthy stories. People who are constantly seeking news items will very much appreciate receiving work that is already half done. If it is interesting, they will help you make it go viral.

Very few things have such a positive impact for your clinic as the publication of an article about your business. In addition, anything in the news is free advertising. Articles are more effective than adverts because the latter, besides costing money, are clearly marketing material.

Ensure they talk about you in a positive light and create a press release. There is a special art to writing press releases, but you can find a lot of online courses if you wish to learn.

It is important to discern between newsworthy facts and those which are not. These are known as criteria of newsworthiness, of which there are three main points:

- Timeliness, because your news must be related to a current hot topic.
- Proximity, because the article affects your area or the people in your vicinity.
- Prominence, a news item featuring a well-known person has more impact.

If you think you have a piece of newsworthy information, proceed with your press release. Offer it to your media contacts.

EXERCISE

Search the internet for journalists committed to animal welfare and get in touch with them. Have an item ready for them.

Social media for millennials

Facebook or the power of recommendation

Facebook is basically the new word-of-mouth. It publishes all sorts of news and information as well as adverts specifically selected for you and your clients. In 2018, Facebook users are better segmented than those of Google, so buying adverts on Facebook is more fruitful than placing them with the "all-powerful search engine". Your adverts are shown exclusively to your target audience, those who have revealed an interest in pets and live in your area.

Think about it for a moment – who do your clients pay the most attention to, a friend or a veterinary surgeon? Maybe we are the exception, but many of our clients place more value on what their friends tell them than the words of a vet. Take advantage of this by getting them to recommend you. Actively invite them to urge their friends to "like" your Facebook page.

Every year, Facebook adds new functions which you can use to entertain your clients: competitions, events, offers, games, shared interest groups. There are many ways to connect sincerely with your clients.

TIP

We have taken it for granted that you have your personal profile on one side and your clinic's profile on the other. It is better to separate your professional and personal lives. Otherwise, if you do not make this distinction, nor will your clients and they will regard you as their friend, with the consequent risk implied if all your clients become friends.

Adding #Hashtags to everything you write will facilitate publishing your messages on other social media. After all, it only takes a second and is very helpful.

Use your Facebook page to send traffic to your website, do not forget to include your website address on the Fanpage* information tab.

EXERCISE

Create your Facebook business page with your monthly cover photo and invite your clients to "like" it. If you only have a few followers, send an email to your emailing lists and invite them to follow you on Facebook.

*A Business Page is a social network tool that Facebook created to allow companies or businesspeople to design and develop marketing campaigns.

The clinic's social media

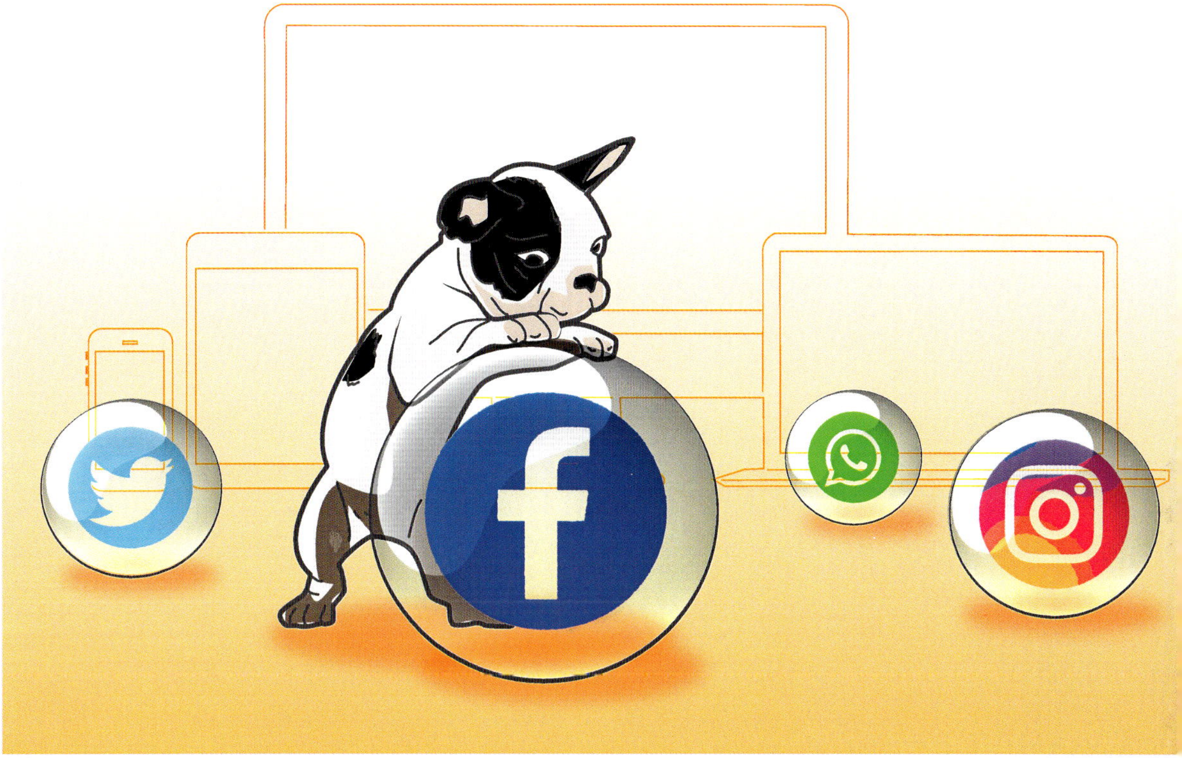

Instant messaging

They are here to stay: WhatsApp, Snapchat, and Telegram are some examples of client communication channels and, like it or not, our clients want us to be available and easily contacted.

Their use does not have to infringe on your daily life if you establish some simple rules. For example, make it clear that WhatsApp is only available during opening hours and is switched off when you close the clinic. In a 24-hour clinic, it offers another means of communication for making appointments or following up.

The only reason to forego the use of instant messaging is because you do not have enough time or a receptionist at the clinic. If that is your case, maybe you should consider hiring someone.

EXERCISE

You are either in or out.

Open WhatsApp to your clients, they will appreciate it.

Power to the image

Maybe you are not part of the millennial generation, but a lot of your clients are, and they live on Instagram or Pinterest. Although you may not be hooked on these networks and those which will emerge in the future, you should be aware of them and publish on them occasionally. Schedule it in your editorial calendar.

From a neuromarketing point of view, images are mightier than text and videos more powerful than photographs, but if you want to win over your clients you should practice storytelling – make a video in which you tell a story.

Play with browsers' curiosity. Curiosity, as explained by neuromarketing, derives from confidence. We investigate because we feel secure, we wouldn't try to discover new things if we felt afraid. From security we develop curiosity, and this takes the mind to another level. For example, set up a competition to determine the breed of a puppy by posting a photo of just a part of its face, then gradually expand the photo until the entire face is visible.

Humour is very effective because it creates bonds and memories. Jokes often start with a known situation that later takes on an unexpected and surprising twist. That is why people like funny animal videos or comic strips. Nevertheless, you must be very careful because the internet has its own rules and you are a veterinary surgeon. Never ridicule or laugh at someone else's misfortune.

EXERCISE

Create an Instagram account and use it to improve the photos taken with your mobile, then upload them to your favourite social media sites. Thus, you can publish two things with just one action. Always add a #Hashtag.

What about LinkedIn?

If you are a specialist vet, you will benefit from a LinkedIn profile. LinkedIn is a professional network that can be used to search for work or potential employees. You can discuss your clinic and include your website on your personal profile.

EXERCISE

Decide whether you need a LinkedIn profile, whether it is worth the extra effort.

Zombie social media

Why do some social media channels succeed, while others fail? They often fail because they do not know why they exist, which could also happen with your clinic. Many have already disappeared or lost millions of users, such as Myspace, and the same thing could happen to others including Twitter and Google +, because their purpose is not very clear.

Twitter can help you keep abreast of the latest news, but if you follow a lot of people, you must pay close attention to avoid missing anything. Therefore, anything you publish on Twitter will only last a short time unless you repeat it several times a day, which is a lot of extra work for very little reward. Google + is useful because Google says so, but it is unclear whether it has any other, as yet unseen, function.

In both cases, they are of little use to promote your veterinary practice because nobody knows why they were created, what they are used for, and therefore they are zombies – the living dead.

EXERCISE

Do not spend too much time and effort with zombie social media. If you already have a profile, just copy content published in your other channels.

Material you should not publish

After discussing the material that makes relevant content and when and where to publish it, we must now talk about the information which is unsuitable for sharing with the public.

Explicit images and scientific texts

It is hard to avoid the temptation to post images of a successful operation that lifted your self-esteem due to its complexity, or a photo of a particularly nasty bite that is curing very well, but most people find these images rather unsightly.

You are not publishing for other vets, so refrain from posting any unpleasant images and texts with lots of veterinary jargon. Preferably your content should be nice to look at and, above all, readable and understandable. Your readers will not understand a comment such as "The problem lies in the coronoid process of the right forelimb", it is better to say "The animal's right elbow hurts."

Do not underestimate mirror neurons: we feel what we see. The sight of blood arouses pain or fear, and clients feel like the dog undergoing surgery in the photo is theirs. Can you imagine your doctor publishing your operation on the internet? I don't think you would appreciate it if your child's paediatrician posted photos of them performing surgery on your son or daughter.

EXERCISE

Revise each text before publishing it and rewrite any overly technical terms using more straightforward words that your non-veterinary friends would understand.

Nonconstructive criticism

Veterinary surgeons are open to public opinion; receiving occasional criticism is part of our work. Consequently, you must react with humility and accept that you can do things better. Sometimes criticism is only designed to ensure you do not repeat an action that upset a specific client. In other cases, the client wants to make a fuss or receive a refund, but you must still respond politely and correctly.

Always try to discuss any incidents in private at the clinic, to avoid creating bad publicity on the internet. While advances are being made regarding the prosecution of crime and defamation on the internet, if someone stirs up trouble for your clinic, the damage will already be done even if attempts are made to repair it later.

EXERCISE

If you receive a complaint or claim against you, invite the client to your clinic so you may listen to what they have to say and offer them a reasonable solution. React calmly and listen carefully, try to put yourself in their position.

Do not swamp your clients with offers

I know this has been said earlier, but it is an important point. This applies to all social media channels (apart from adverts, of course). Do not post more than one commercial offer among every four informative items you publish on social media.

Online reputation

There is a popular saying that in Chinese, the word "crisis" is composed of two characters. One means "danger", while the other is "opportunity".

> "In a crisis, be aware of the danger – but recognise the opportunity."
> *John F. Kennedy*

You can work your fingers to the bone and obtain clients who are in love with your clinic, but suddenly one person criticises your work and all your effort is undermined. Times have changed, in the past, this unsatisfied client would voice their complaint/slander in the park and 10 people would hear it, regardless of whether it was true; now they complain through the internet and negative points have a stronger impact than positive ones, so you must be prepared.

How to deal with a crisis 3.0

Firstly, you must determine whether the crisis situation is due to a complaint from an unsatisfied client or in response to an unfortunate error by the community manager. If, on the other hand, the situation is based on the actions of a troll*, the best thing to do is just ignore it. However, if the complaint is genuine, well-founded, and casts doubt on the company's reputation, either because of an inappropriate publication or a client's dissatisfaction, the community manager must act rapidly by implementing a previously established action protocol, which should be common to all clinics. Waiting for a problem to arise before deciding how to act is a serious error that could cost your company a lot of followers.

EXERCISE

Draft your crisis management protocol. We shall help you a little.

CRISIS MANAGEMENT PROTOCOL

First of all, you must be prepared:

1. Select the staff member who will implement the protocol. It is important that you know who should be informed of the crisis, the key person who will take decisions about how to resolve it, and where to find them at all times. Crises do not wait until 9 o'clock on Monday morning before erupting.
2. Permanent monitoring. Paying attention to any warning signals on SM sites is essential for detecting the crisis as early as possible and tackling it without risking your company's reputation.
3. Risk assessment. Respond or leave it unanswered? Should you reassert your argument or agree with the client? At this point your clinic must state its position very clearly in each case, while always distinguishing between genuine complaints and malicious allegations from trolls.
4. Develop a crisis action plan.

*Troll: in this context, a troll is someone who publishes inflammatory messages with the sole intention of bothering others and creating confrontation either for their own amusement or financial reasons, such as a competitor who wants to be a nuisance.

At the onset of the crisis: listen/act/respond/address/neutralise

1. It is imperative that you listen to the public to learn what the problem is, to discover what is causing the crisis.
2. Remain calm. Being too hasty never helps, particularly in stressful situations where your clinic's reputation is on the line.
3. Try to resolve the problem. If only one person has made the complaint, try to deal with it in private through direct messages. In most cases, this is generally enough to smooth the waters, reach an agreement with the client, and close the case.
4. Use a polite tone and language.
5. Do not censor negative comments. The worst mistake you can make when managing a crisis is to delete the message that triggered the problem, as it will only fuel the client's anger further. Nor is it a good idea to delete the message when the crisis concerns content published by the brand, unless the comment is offensive or blatantly violates the company's ideology.
6. In the event of an error, admit the fault and apologise.
7. Provide a clear and accurate explanation through a press release, the company website, and/or the social media channels where you have a presence.
8. Never respond in the heat of the moment.

During the crisis: react/respond/reconsider

1. Make the case a priority. Do not avoid it, follow up on the complaint. It is the most important thing you need to deal with today and over the next few days.
2. Try to defuse the crisis, make sure it does not escalate. See to it that the client knows their complaint is being studied and you are dealing with it personally, so they will receive a rapid solution or response.

3. If the crisis gives rise to more online complaints, reduce the visibility of the negative comments, but do not censor or delete any of them. Remember, if the comment only intends to cause trouble, do not reply.
4. Show the unsatisfied person that you are keen to resolve their problem.
5. Avoid ambiguous messages.
6. If you are subject to an unfounded or slanderous attack, discuss it with your lawyer.

After the crisis: recover/learn/protect

1. Assess the consequences of the crisis.
2. Analyse whether you have correctly followed the procedures defined in your crisis management protocol.
3. Decide whether you should modify the clinic's internal communication procedures.
4. Check if the crisis has destabilised the company, if you have lost followers, and analyse the current status of your online reputation (and even your offline reputation in severe cases).
5. Investigate whether your company has been discussed in SM channels where you previously had no presence. If so, open an account on these platforms to clear your reputation.

Once you have overcome the crisis, your best option is to seek new positive comments to replace the negative ones. You have three main lines of action:

- YouTube testimonials. It is the perfect moment to upload new testimonials to your channel.
- Reviews in Google. Ask your best clients to post a rating on Google.
- Facebook opinions. Everyone receives a few negative comments, but you will have greater credibility if the majority are positive. If all the users give you a 5-star rating, they are clearly your friends. A rating of 4.5 appears more trustworthy and genuine than a score of 5.0.

SUMMARY

- Your social media strategy is more important than which channels you use. SM can change, but you should use a similar neuromarketing sales strategy, adapting yourself to the new platforms.
- Set aside half a day per week for you, or the person responsible but under your supervision, to work on your SM.
- Dedicate a fraction of your monthly revenue to internet advertising. Normally, 1 % is enough, although you can invest more and more efficiently with professional help.
- Take photos and videos on a daily basis and upload them to favourite your social media site. You can touch them up with Instagram or a similar application.
- Develop your personal brand and differential value proposition (DVP).
- Define your ideal client, the person your messages will focus on.
- Design your editorial calendar and identify the social media channels where you want to have an active presence. Schedule your publications and select one of your team to help share the duties of the community manager.
- Once a month, spend a morning or afternoon writing the content you scheduled in your editorial calendar. You will only have to publish it when the time comes.
- Review and update your website, open a social media account and create your blog. Design your cover photos/banners.
- Don't sell, inform. The aim is to build loyalty. Share interesting content, both your own and third-party content. You can obtain it from Google Alerts and Google Trends.
- Post short, punchy texts and always add a #Hashtag. Videos are better than photos, but they should always tell us a story.
- Testimonials are very powerful tools, both written and video endorsements.
- Create your clinic's digital crisis management protocol. If you are prepared, you will know how to react appropriately.

14 Neuromarketing over the telephone

Your telephone service is a central pillar of your veterinary clinic's communication.

The ten most important benefits of attending the telephone correctly

1 Many new clients will first contact your clinic through this channel. The rate of defections or dropouts (the churn rate) is close to 45 % in the veterinary sector. Therefore, survival is only feasible for veterinary practices if they can attract new pet owners to maintain or increase their number of active clients. Calls help prevent and reduce the number of desertions.

The telephone is a source of income.

2 The telephone is a powerful weapon for earning the loyalty of clients who have already visited your clinic. A call from the veterinary surgeon to ask how a patient is doing the day after their operation, or to follow up on a clinical case, is a pleasant surprise that cements your bond with the client and portrays professionalism and quality treatment.

3 It is a potent, efficient, and cost-effective tool for issuing appointment reminders, besides being most clients' preferred means of communication compared to letters or emails.

4 The telephone is also useful for recovering clients who have stopped using your services or missed an appointment. You can discover why they have left your clinic or if they have simply forgotten their scheduled appointments. To do this you need a good CRM (customer relationship management) system or tools that can segment clients who are purchasing or using your services less often or detect ones who have deserted your clinic (i.e. those who have not used your services in the past year).

5 It represents the client's voice. The telephone can be used to carry out service quality or client satisfaction surveys. The staff member who will conduct the survey must discuss and agree on the questions, their purpose, and the means of measuring the marketing results with the rest of the team before making the calls. All calls should be logged in a standardised register to ensure employees making the calls follow a protocol and the validity of the quality survey as a basis for subsequent decisions. Satisfaction surveys not only provide an evaluation of the quality of your veterinary services, but they also help reveal your real needs, not just the ones you presume to know or suspect as a vet.

Any telephone surveys you design should always be clearly focused on assessing the quality of service and the client's needs and preferences.

6 Share all the information you gather, organise, and finally evaluate with the rest of the team, so they also get involved in the areas for improvement. Similarly, you should clarify the methodology used to measure the results, as we shall see in the more detailed explanation of the NPS method given in Chapter 5.

7 The telephone can also be used as a communication tool for disseminating marketing campaigns. This needs to be based on a good segmentation of clients; you do not want to call clients with puppies and offer them products or services for elderly dogs, for example. A comprehensive software package for all staff, such as SuiteCRM, would be particularly useful.

Calls to VIP clients: you must treat these clients with special, preferential attention because they provide 80 % of your revenue. According to the Pareto principle, 20 % of clients generate 80 % of a business' income. In a well-managed veterinary clinic this proportion of the best clients is closer to 30 %. Use these calls to offer additional or complementary services.

8 Frequency of calls: be careful to avoid making too many or too few calls. In the case of clients who visit your practice often, you only need call to check on their pet's clinical progress. Whereas calling infrequent visitors would help obtain new appointments.

9 Inform or communicate? Information is the one-way message you sent out from the clinic. On the other hand, communication is a message that relies on a feedback loop. In terms of client satisfaction and the clinic–client relationship, you should create a communicative link. Although the call is initially placed to provide information, the conversation with the client should be interactive and fluid.

When communicating, you must bear in mind the goals you are trying to achieve:

- Modify a behaviour: for example, increase the number of repeat purchases or promote a new service.
- Consolidate a behaviour: maintain the level of client loyalty.
- Gather information: find out why the client does not use, for example, the pet grooming service, or where they purchase flea collars.

Customer value proposition (CVP): the conversation must revolve around issues that address the clients' needs or which are value drivers.

The number of telephone calls your clinic receives is a direct indicator of the business' health.

Also remember that the telephone can be used to send WhatsApp messages, images, and videos, as we shall see later in this chapter.

Before answering a call

We have already stressed the importance of making a good first impression, which is even more crucial on the telephone because this channel lacks the support of background noises or the visual cues available during face-to-face exchanges. That is why you must learn to master this tool.

An appropriate greeting

Whoever answers the phone transmits the company and brand image, and the client will make their own personal evaluation of the attention they receive. If you treat the client politely, they will view the clinic as respectful, and if you empathise with them, it will create a mental image of good professionals.

Always maintain a smile

We can detect when someone is smiling over the phone. What is more, humans can differentiate between genuine and forced smiles. The face takes on a distinct shape depending on whether or not it is smiling, which makes the voice sound different.

Do not speed up while speaking

You should speak 20 % slower than normal. Furthermore, always make sure you articulate very clearly for older clients.

Attending the phone

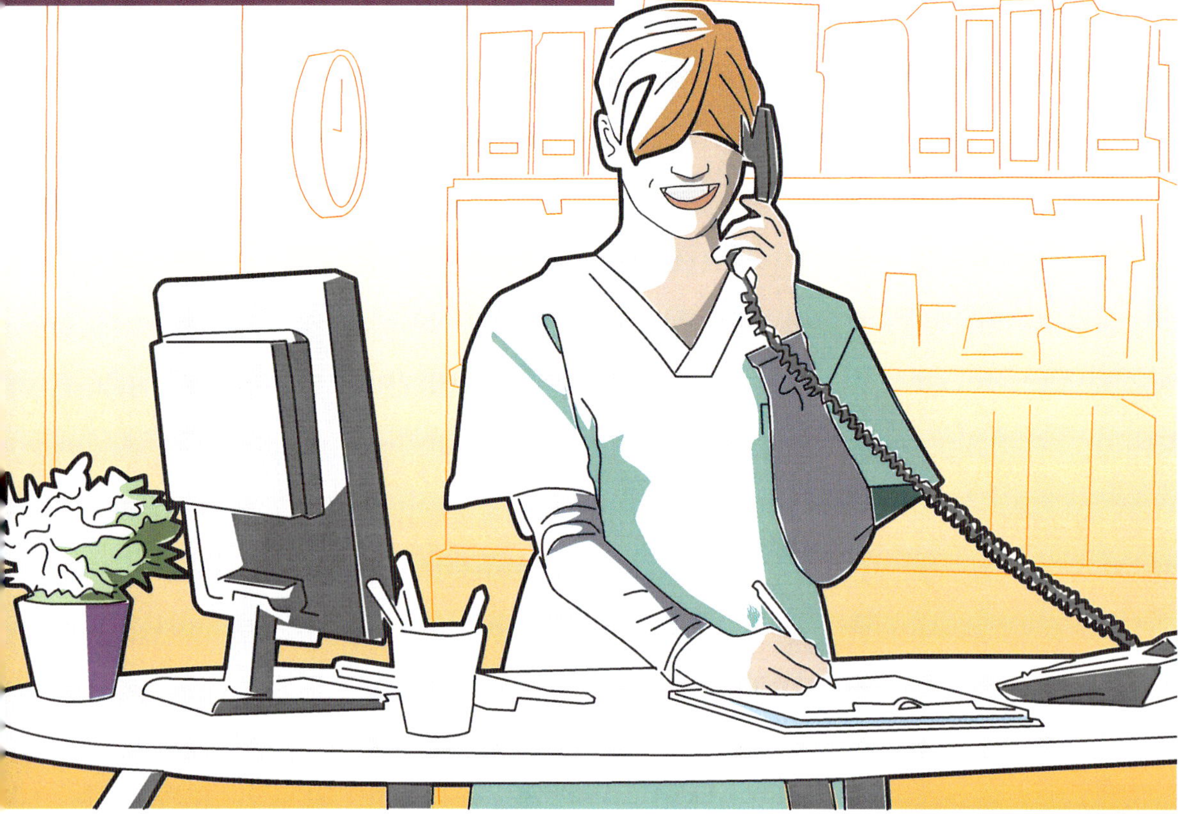

Paralanguage is important

Make use of paralanguage, that is, all the sounds that we use to emphasise what you are saying or that you are listening actively. For instance, when someone is telling you what has happened to them, you must show that you are interested and truly listening. Sounds of agreement such as "uh-huh" and "hmm" are advisable.

Empathy is obligatory

It is important to empathise with the client. The best thing to do is find something in common and strike up a conversation about it; ask what their pet is called, its breed, if they have any children, etc., these questions are easy to formulate and make the subsequent conversation about the pet's problem flow more smoothly.

Never forget to say "thank you"

After arranging an appointment or before hanging up, always thank the client and remind them who you are. If you have just organised an appointment, you could tell them where to find the nearest car park or send them the clinic's location via WhatsApp. Before finishing the call, you should have adhered to the "CAT" rule and arranged to speak with the client again through any of the options listed below.

THE "CAT" RULE

- Call
- Appointment
- Text message (reminder)

In the client's mind, each of these aspects will be subconsciously associated with the quality of the service and veterinary attention.

Using language

Avoid using overly technical language on the telephone. Use straightforward, comprehensible language.

Points of interest

The staff member who answers the call must determine if it is a veterinary emergency. They must be trained and used to formulating questions about basic details such as:

- For how long has the animal been unwell?
- What is their breathing like?
- Do they have a fever?
- Is the animal coughing or in pain?
- Are they happy and active or motionless and sad?

If you think it is an emergency, get in touch with the veterinary surgeon and offer an immediate appointment.

Sometimes what the client considers to be an emergency does not meet the applicable clinical criteria. You can resolve this problem by creating the concepts of priority calls or appointments, which indicates it is an emergency situation for the owner but not the pet, and emergency appointments, which are genuinely life-threatening situations. The whole team must be very clear on the difference.

ONLY EVER USE NEGATIVE WORDS WITH GREAT CARE

What you might say...	What you ought to say...
We cannot.	We shall try to.
I don't know.	I shall look for the information and call you back this afternoon.
The vet cannot attend you at the moment.	Please give me your phone number and we will do everything we can to call you between 5 and 6 pm.
I cannot diagnose your pet's illness over the phone.	Your case is very interesting, and the vet can fit you in this afternoon at 5 pm, would you like me to book an appointment for you? What you have just told me seems very important. Someone has just cancelled an appointment this afternoon at 6 pm, is that a good time for you to bring Shep?
We cannot provide an estimate for a knee operation without seeing the patient.	We can give you an estimate this afternoon if you bring all the X-rays, laboratory test results, and your pet to the clinic for an examination. The trauma specialist will explain the different types of solutions available for your pet. Would an appointment at 6 pm suit you?
We cannot see you today, we are very busy.	Someone has just cancelled an appointment for tomorrow at 11 am, would you like me to reserve that slot for you?
The vet cannot come to the phone, I have already interrupted him three times.	Tell me what's worrying you so that I may help.

Phrases such as "I shall try to slot you in at X o'clock", or "I will look after Bobby until the vet is available to take care of him" can be particularly helpful when dealing with owners who are worried about noncritical emergencies.

Standard telephone protocol

1. Take a deep breath and smile.
2. Presentation: the company and person who answers the call.
3. Offer to help.
4. Listen to the client.
5. Look for a common point.
6. Ask about the exact nature of their concern (sometimes the client does not know how to explain the real problem and they mention a secondary one).
7. Try to find a solution by offering an appointment. You can say the vet has a full agenda, but there is a slot at X o'clock; the principle of scarcity will urge the owner to accept the time on offer.
8. Schedule the appointment and take note of all the details.

Offering an appointment

You should try to fill those gaps in the agenda that tend to appear in the early morning or on slow days. Consequently, you should always offer these slots before others, but while accommodating the client's availability. Firstly, ask whether the client prefers mornings or afternoons. After confirming their preference, ask them to choose either an early or late appointment. The next step is to offer two options within their chosen period, from among the slots you would like to fill. If you ask the client when is convenient for them but this slot is already reserved, it will be harder to agree a time.

Giving estimates over the phone

In 90 % of cases the price is the excuse for starting up a conversation and often for arranging an initial examination, but 10 % of calls are only made to enquire about prices and estimates. Nevertheless, you should still give them your full attention because they may call again later and eventually show an interest in the clinic. People call because they want to form an opinion about your centre.

Finding a common link is straightforward. For example, if someone brings in a puppy, ask them what breed it is, or say something like "Aww, what a cute little thing", "I had a Westie", "What is his name?", or "Why did you choose that name?" There are many questions you can use to approach the person.

The important point is to find a common link with the client.

Do not forget the aim of the call is to arrange an appointment and, where possible, fill out their record over the phone. If they request an estimate, the first thing to do is explain the work involved, what the procedure or operation entails. It is worth asking if they have discussed it with another veterinary surgeon as maybe their vet does not offer this service, or perhaps they prefer the operation to be performed in a better-equipped clinic or which has been recommended by another pet owner. If they tell you why, record all the information, give them a rough estimate and then try to arrange an appointment. Although it is better to give an appointment and later explain the estimate at the clinic, not all owners are prepared to invest their time without being told the estimate.

You must explain the benefits the procedure offers for their pet: the incisions are small, they will stay in heated incubators during hospitalisation, animals are monitored at all times, early spaying eliminates the chances of mammary tumours, etc.

Equally, you must point out the advantages for the owner: they can drop off their animal in the morning and collect them after lunch, they can pay with a credit card, postoperative checkups and stitch removal are included in the price, the animal will be examined and tests conducted before surgery, their pet will feel much better after the procedure and receive close monitoring, they will receive a video of Bobby as soon as he wakes up, there is no need to worry, etc. You must help the owner visualise the entire treatment process and the advantages they will obtain with your clinic compared to others, so the client feels confident and relaxed about the situation.

Another important point is to avoid talking badly about other vets as it gives off a very bad image. In response to a claim that your prices are high you could say: "I do not know how they perform this procedure in other centres, but I can explain how we do it here and you can decide", or "For your peace of mind, we can show you our facilities and fully equipped operating theatre, so you can see how sterile and safe everything is for your pet."

Do not forget that the information you provide during the call is the first step in the loyalty-building procedure.

Handling complaints over the phone

You should handle telephone complaints following the same protocol as those made in person:

- Firstly, let the client speak and vent their irritation without interrupting them.
- Secondly, tell the client you understand their point of view.
- Thirdly, ask them if they would like to receive a call from the team member implicated in the complaint, in which they will try to offer a solution.

It is particularly important that you adhere to the agreed timing of events. If you told the client the vet would call them at 2 pm, then you must fulfil this promise.

Everyone in the team must agree on the complaint status monitoring system. You should categorise complaints into groups.

Closed complaint

With four possible results:

- Only favourable for the client.
- Favourable for the client and the company.
- Unfavourable.
- Very unfavourable.

Active complaint: an unresolved situation

- In the process of being resolved, without having yet reached an agreement between the client and clinic.
- In the hands of the courts, when one or both parties have filed a complaint and it is pending a decision.
- Final ruling but pending execution.
- Payment order procedure pending collection.

Having said this, all complaints, whether justified or not, must be dealt with quickly and individually.

In cases where the complaint is justified, you must always start by apologising and following the initial protocol.

Use plain language in your response and avoid technical terms, and never make any promises that you cannot fulfil. Finally, at the end of the conversation, conclude by thanking the client for getting in touch with the clinic and helping improve your service.

An ideal target would be to resolve 75 % of complaints during the first interaction with the client.

Monitor your telephone service

To monitor the telephone service you provide and ensure improvement processes are implemented correctly, we recommend you:

- Measure the number of incoming calls compared to appointments made, giving you a prospective client conversion ratio.
- Keep a record of calls so you can follow up on animals after surgery and those receiving ongoing treatment. It is advisable to use the agenda for this task.
- Conduct client recovery campaigns over the phone. List names, the date of the call, and the clients recovered by this channel.
- Maintain an agenda for reminders of upcoming appointments.

The telephone as a communication tool

The way we use the telephone has changed a lot since the turn of the century. The possibility of taking photographs and videos with mobile phones has facilitated better communication with clients and improved loyalty-building, recuperation, and patient acquisition. When used correctly, the telephone bears a direct influence on a clinic's balance sheet.

Explaining what an operation involves or sending a photograph of a recovering patient after an intervention are tools with a strong emotional impact on the client. Such actions form part of their perception of veterinary and human quality. If your clients perform searches with their telephones, or use them to record their pets, then as a vet, you can use them in a similar manner to further your clinic's interests.

The use of WhatsApp, email, or mobile apps portrays an up-to-date image in terms of new technologies and therefore your veterinary services will also emanate a modern, cutting-edge appearance.

WhatsApp, however, can also act as a double-edged sword, so you must use it with care. It is a good tool for communicating with clients who are abroad, thus reducing costs for both parties. Nevertheless, you must think carefully about what you write as it will remain in the client's phone, and if you do not fulfil any promises or prognoses, the messages could be used against you by a lawyer. For example, if you write "Don't worry nothing will happen, your animal's situation is not serious", and the pet subsequently dies, well you could be facing a major problem.

You should hold a meeting with your team to draw up a WhatsApp usage protocol and explain the risks of improper use. Ensure you all refrain from giving diagnoses, treatment guidelines, or prognoses. Therefore, WhatsApp can prove to be a very useful tool for managing appointments and maintaining customer loyalty, but strictly avoid messages regarding clinical information.

Return on investment (ROI)

You must always weigh up expenditure in terms of human resources, in other words, compare the effective cost of time spent by auxiliary personnel when making these calls against the resulting tangible and intangible benefits. So before carrying out a telephone campaign you must consider its predicted percentage of effectiveness and the benefits it will produce in terms of revenue (tangible) and quality (intangible).

POINTS TO REMEMBER WHEN ON THE TELEPHONE

- Your goal is to convert calls into appointments.
- It is advisable to have several lines, so clients do not have to wait. The phone should never ring more than three times before someone answers.
- Never give out false information or false expectations. If a client requests some information that is not available at that time, tell them you will make sure it reaches them as soon as it is available.
- When you commit to a date to respond to a query, you must abide by the promised timeline. These details are associated with professionalism and reliability.
- Schedule calls into the vet's agenda so they have enough time to respond to outstanding queries: "The vet will call you back between 2:00 and 2:20 this afternoon." The client will be pleasantly surprised if the vet calls earlier than expected.

15 Using neuromarketing to manage critical points during consultations

Difficult moments often arise at the clinic, we are all familiar with them and staff fear these incidents because they cannot always handle them correctly, yet they are critical to the future of a business, as they may have a strong influence on whether the client revisits the practice. Examples include how you address euthanasia, respond to a complaint, receive payment for your services, deal with a crisis of reputation on social media, etc.

To manage these situations correctly you must establish some protocols, so instead of improvising you can apply a previously concocted "recipe" that is specific to each case.

We suggest you write your own protocols for each situation after reading this chapter.

Dealing with loss: when euthanasia becomes necessary

Sometimes, after a long relationship with a veterinary practice, the vet may manage an animal's euthanasia poorly. If this happens, the owner may not want to return with a new pet because their last visit was too painful.

Pain creates a long-term memory in the primitive brain, so you must handle this type of situation with extreme sensitivity.

There is a story and a family behind each animal. Never downplay the importance of this moment in a person's life.

Points to consider:

- All staff must be aware when a patient is going to visit the clinic for this procedure, especially those in reception, so they can use language befitting of the occasion.
- It is a good idea to suggest that the owner brings someone else with them.

- Ensure there are no background noises such as staff laughing or chatting during the process, you must be highly respectful of other people's pain.
- Do not leave the client alone in reception where they can hear other clients' conversations or may be asked to explain their visit.
- Ideally, you should arrange an appointment, so they do not have to wait; either early in the morning, before opening, or at the end of the day, to respect their intimacy and the pain caused by the loss.
- Prepare a room for the process, but do not use the main consultation room, where possible, so the client does not have to revisit this space if they return with another pet. It must be an isolated room, without passage to another area.
- Explain the process with a calm voice. Factors such as sedation, the act of euthanasia, and incineration must be explained clearly.
- The owner must sign an informed consent form before the procedure. Where possible, prepare the subject of payment, which you must introduce tactfully. If it is very awkward, given the tension of the moment, you can leave it until the end of the visit in reception.
- Ask the owner if they wish to accompany their pet throughout the process.
- Children and individuals in poor health or in delicate situations are advised not to attend the procedure, and you should inform the owner about this point.
- If these people insist on attending, it helps if you have prepared disclaimer forms, so they may sign them and assume responsibility for any problems that could arise, both medical and psychological.
- You must explain the grieving process to the people who accompany the owner.

If the client gets angry: complaints

In this chapter we will deal with complaints made in person, as we already discussed complaints over the telephone in a previous chapter.

Points to consider:

- Remove the person from the waiting room and take them to a more private room. When there is an audience, like in reception, arguments can become heated and the person complaining may feel their position is substantiated.
- Ease the tension; let them speak and present their complaint. People with a complaint often create an internal dialogue in which they imagine discussing and arguing with their counterpart. Allowing them to speak uninterrupted will help them relax.
- Your body language should express agreement and active listening. Look the client in the eyes and relax your body. Assure them you are listening by tilting your head to one side as this transmits interest.

USING PARALANGUAGE IN CASES OF EUTHANASIA

The vet's body does not have to be particularly erect.

They can touch the people who accompany the animal as a sign of affection and proximity. People pick up on this empathy under these circumstances and it is very important they do not feel alone.

You should indicate that you understand the pain with phrases such as "I know this is a very hard moment", or "We're sorry you have to go through this."

You could say the animal was lucky to have had such a full life and will not have to suffer anymore.

Allow enough time for the farewell and silent moments. Do not rush the client.

When they leave the clinic, a firm handshake or placing your hand lightly on their right shoulder is a sign of proximity and empathy.

If it is a large animal, never drag them or place them in a bag when the client is present. The animal remains asleep and you can finish the process when the client has left.

We recommend either calling the client or sending them a letter of condolence approximately a week after the event.

- If they are using aggressive body language or shouting, you must reply politely and with a quiet voice. They should never be disrespectful or intimidate any of your staff.
- After the complainant has explained their grievance, tell them you understand how they feel.
- Sometimes the client has just cause to complain and you may have committed a mistake. Admitting this fact and offering a sincere apology could help a lot, as people do not expect such a response. It is one way of proposing a better solution to the problem.
- If there is a means of resolving the complaint, you must commit to a solution and time limit.
- However, if you believe the complaint is unjustified, you must explain your opinion calmly.
- You must not give in to blackmail.
- If the complaint is due to bad service or an excessively long wait, you must endeavour to speak with the person responsible so that it does not happen again.

- You must always thank the client for the information because it does not always reach you. The mere fact that the complainant has entered your clinic to discuss the matter means they want a personal response and are involved in the process.

The awkward moment of payment

Veterinary surgeons often feel uncomfortable when it comes to receiving payment. This is further compounded by the fact that payment equates to a loss for the client and you must try to minimise this effect.

The sense of loss is greater when paying in cash.

That is why paying with smartphones or deferred payment options are so successful, as the loss is less tangible when using credit cards. Consumers tend to fall into more debt when using these methods because the purchaser does not experience such a strong sense of loss.

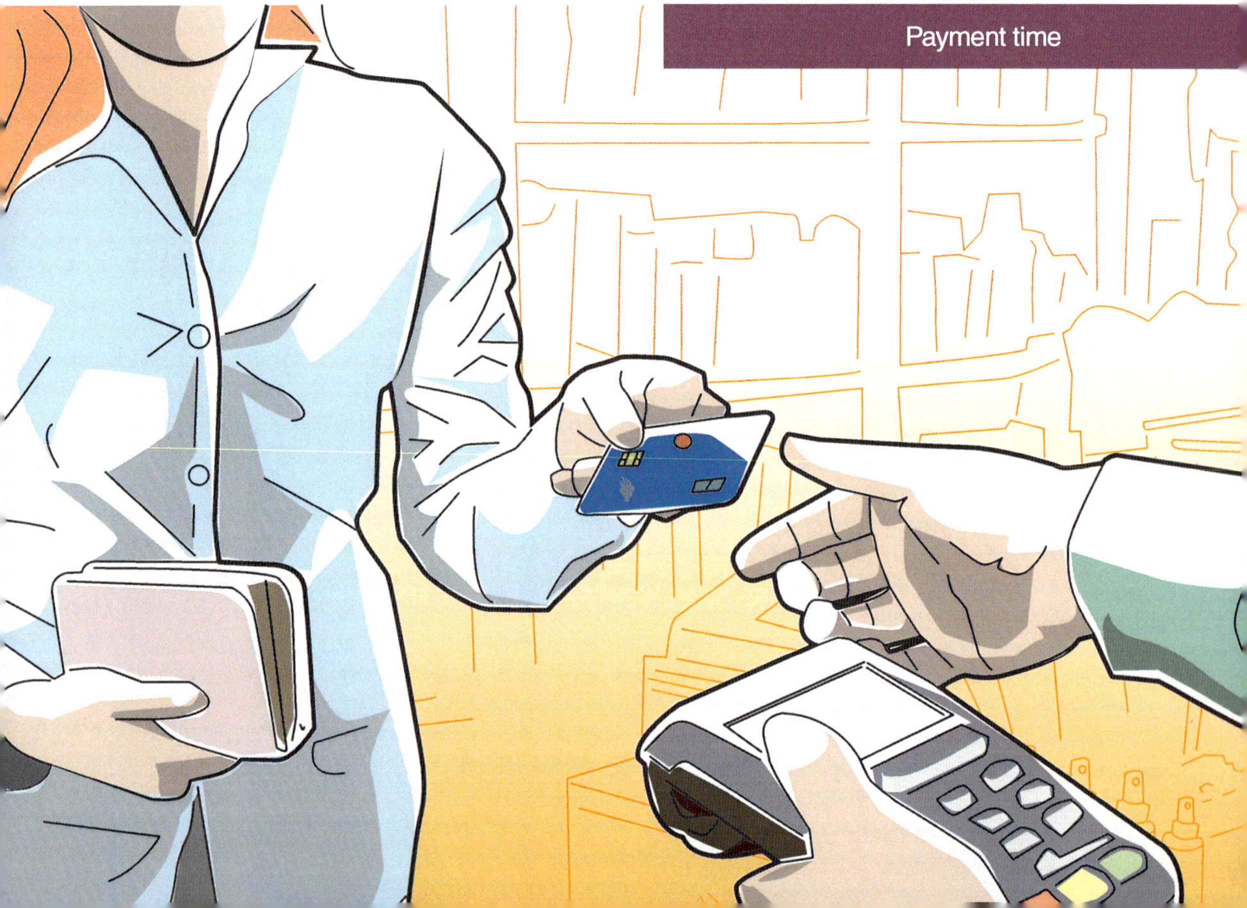

Payment time

However, there is another method to minimise the pain associated with spending money; by making the client appreciate what they receive in return and conclude that it is worth the cost.

This can be achieved by generating pleasure at the time of payment through actions such as:

- Offering the client chocolate or sweets. Eating chocolate produces pleasure and diminishes any tension during payment.
- Soft music to make the process more pleasurable.
- Whilst they are paying, tell a story about the benefits the client will derive. You could say "We hope Bobby will be back to his old self in a few days" to create a positive image in the consumer's mind.
- You can reinforce the feeling of belonging to a special group by mentioning how lucky Bobby is to have such an owner. Many other people are not as committed to looking after their pets.
- Thank the client for their effort and remark how lucky Bobby is.

How to rescue a crisis of reputation

Something as innocent as clicking a "Like" on a Facebook page can result in a bigger headache than you can imagine. The following example is based on a true story experienced by a colleague who specialises in veterinary dentistry.

Imagine you go to visit your local zoo, to help supervise your son's class on their school trip, and you have a great day. The animals are reasonably well looked after given their habitat, and the children enjoyed the experience, learnt a lot, and some plan to travel to Africa to see them in their natural surroundings. So far, everything is normal.

When you get home, you receive a message asking you to rate your visit to the zoo. You enter the zoo's Facebook page and click on "Like", and within 15 minutes your clinic's Facebook page receives dozens of messages (some from your clients) criticising you for supporting an entity that locks up wild animals under terrible conditions.

Oddly enough, a few days earlier some colleagues from your clinic had to visit the zoo and treat an animal's dental problem; they noted the facilities were in very good order, and the zoo's vets and auxiliary staff who assisted with the operation were very well trained and treated their animals with respect.

WHAT IS THE SOLUTION?

In this case you should proceed as follows:

1. Remove your "Like" from the zoo's Facebook page.
2. Write the following message on your Facebook page: "In response to complaints from clients and friends of our clinic we have decided to remove the "Like" from the zoo's page to show we are against wild animals being held in captivity. However, we would also like to make it known that animals at the zoo receive the best possible veterinary and nutritional care given the circumstances, as we were able to confirm last month when we carried out a dental procedure on a leopard who was experiencing difficulties swallowing."

WHAT DOES THIS GESTURE ACHIEVE?

1. It demonstrates your appreciation of the issue and that you agree with those who complained.
2. It reminds your clients that you are specialists in veterinary dentistry, to such an extent that a zoo requested your help with a very special patient.

WHAT CAN YOU LEARN FROM THIS CASE?

1. Before "Liking" a Facebook page, consider the pros and cons of your action, since you are not acting personally but rather as a company devoted to safeguarding animal health, with everything that it entails.
2. You must react rapidly to any social media "fires" and already have a crisis management protocol in place to help you stay calm and deal with the conflict.

Here is another example of a well-intended action that could end in disaster if managed poorly.

It's 8 pm on Friday and you are about to close the clinic. A client enters with a parrot in a cage that they found abandoned beside a rubbish container and they do not know what to do. The parrot does not have a ring and is in a poor condition, so you trim its beak, prepare a space in the inpatients area, and place it under observation. You leave the clinic late, but happy for carrying out your good deed for the day, or better said one more. You take a photo and post it on Facebook in search of an adoptive owner and, as luck would have it, after 3 days a client comes to adopt the parrot.

Everything seems to have turned out perfectly, hasn't it?

However, the clinic's website starts to receive messages from unknown senders, with animal activist profiles, saying things such as "How can you possibly put an animal up for adoption without performing a blood test and all the other necessary tests, it's a disgrace." As it happens, there was already a cat and a rabbit looking for a home that week, with whom you had done exactly the same; looked after them, treated them, and published their photos on Facebook, but they did not enjoy the same luck as the parrot.

WHAT CAN YOU DO?

1. In this case, which is also based on a true story, the clinic's own clients took the first step by replying to those who had complained in the case of the parrot. They said the clinic had always been very supportive of abandoned animals, as shown by the cases of the cat and rabbit, that they also had a right to find a family, etc. There were so many messages supporting the clinic that the people who complained about the parrot did not write anything else and their comments disappeared from view.
2. What is more, the clinic also stated the parrot would be temporarily sheltered by the adoptive owner for 20 days and, if everything went well, the adoption would become permanent as the bird was perfectly healthy.

WHAT CAN YOU LEARN FROM THIS CASE?

1. Sometimes clients are your best advocates when you have not done anything wrong, they may even help you without having to ask.
2. Always stay calm, act correctly, and communicate.
3. There is no need to delete aggressive comments, as they are discredited by their own merits and other people's replies. Having said that, you can choose to "hide" the comment so the author can still see it but while concealing it from everyone else's view. This is often unnecessary because other comments make it fall down the list and disappear out of sight.

TIP

As a general strategy for dealing with any crisis of reputation, we recommend you post new publications so the ones causing the problem soon become old news. Sometimes it is better to ignore rather than confront the situation; you could present your reasons at first but avoid entering into a long debate as it is better to focus your attention on another issue.

16 Managing internal clients. Employee communication and motivation

Introduction

All veterinary clinics have first-line direct consumers of their services and products, in other words, their administrative and technical teams. Your staff are constantly receiving information about what you have to offer and may want to use your services.

Veterinary clinics are generally small companies where the manager and employees build a close relationship. When staff have a problem regarding their pets' health and routine care they take them to the clinic where they work, but how do your employees handle caring for their pets? Do they have health plans? Do they deworm their pets on a monthly basis? Do they have a correct vaccination programme? Is the clinic owner a role model of suitable pet care and attention?

The idea is to get your internal clients to consume your offers, products, health plans, and prevention plans, then you can receive their feedback to ensure continuous improvement in the implementation of new products. This is the only way your team can develop the skills required to explain and sell the clinic's products, as they will have already tried them. The manager assumes responsibility for equipping the staff with the knowledge and tools they need to promote and justify the services offered by the clinic.

The importance of personality traits and communication

Interpersonal relationships are reciprocal interactions between two or more people. Each employee has a more or less effective ability to communicate with the rest of the team. A knowledge of communication patterns can improve this ability if employees know how to apply it correctly.

There are several methods to identify a team's different personality traits and communication styles, two of the most popular ones are DISC (https://www.discprofile.com/what-is-disc/overview/) and the Myers–Briggs Type Indicator® (MBTI). They all use questionnaires to classify individuals and the overall team into profiles according to their effective and ineffective characteristics when in situations of stress.

The Bridge method describes a group of people who are more rational compared to another, more emotional group. Hence, with respect to communication, we tend to discuss the predominance of one side of the brain.

Rational people (left hemisphere) place greater emphasis on intellect rather than feelings and emotions, so they find it hard to express signs of affection such as hugs and kisses. That is why others may perceive them as aloof or cold. They are motivated by the analysis of data.

This group can be divided into two subgroups:

- **Reflective–rational**. People in this subgroup speak slowly and leave silent pauses while they analyse all the information they receive, like a computer. They are intellectual, focus their attention on thinking, find it hard to express their emotions, and barely use gestures. They tend to talk in theoretical terms and rarely about themselves, they are shy, usually solitary, often perfectionists and attentive in their work, and before they accept a new idea they must be shown that it is feasible. Reflective–rational people are highly organised and annoyed by other people's disorder, which they do not understand. There may be confrontations with the rest of the team because they sometimes seem inflexible, cold, and distrustful. When they feel insecure, the emotion that predominates is fear. They need to feel secure and in control of their environment. They would prefer to play a game of chess before doing physical sport. Interestingly, they often share a particular body shape, that is, they are usually tall and thin.

- **Active–rational**. These people are less intellectual, but similar to the previous subgroup in that they also analyse data. However, they make decisions more quickly, are impatient, energetic, competitive, good at conflict resolution, and assume risks easily. They often talk quickly and get straight to the point. They like starting projects and are very enterprising people. Ineffectiveness may arise from their hasty decision-making and impatience with routine tasks, thus leading to some mistakes. The team may feel uncomfortable because they believe these people do not stop to listen. They like sports and often have an athletic physique. When they feel bad, they are overcome by anger, helplessness, and frustration.

On the other hand, some people are more **emotional** than rational, and normally use more emotive vocabulary. Their right hemispheres are said to predominate. Physically, they usually have wider, rounder faces and display affection and warmth more easily through hugs and kisses. They are often affected by what other people say. Emotional people predominantly feel sad. They sometimes confuse empathy with friendliness.

Rational and emotional people

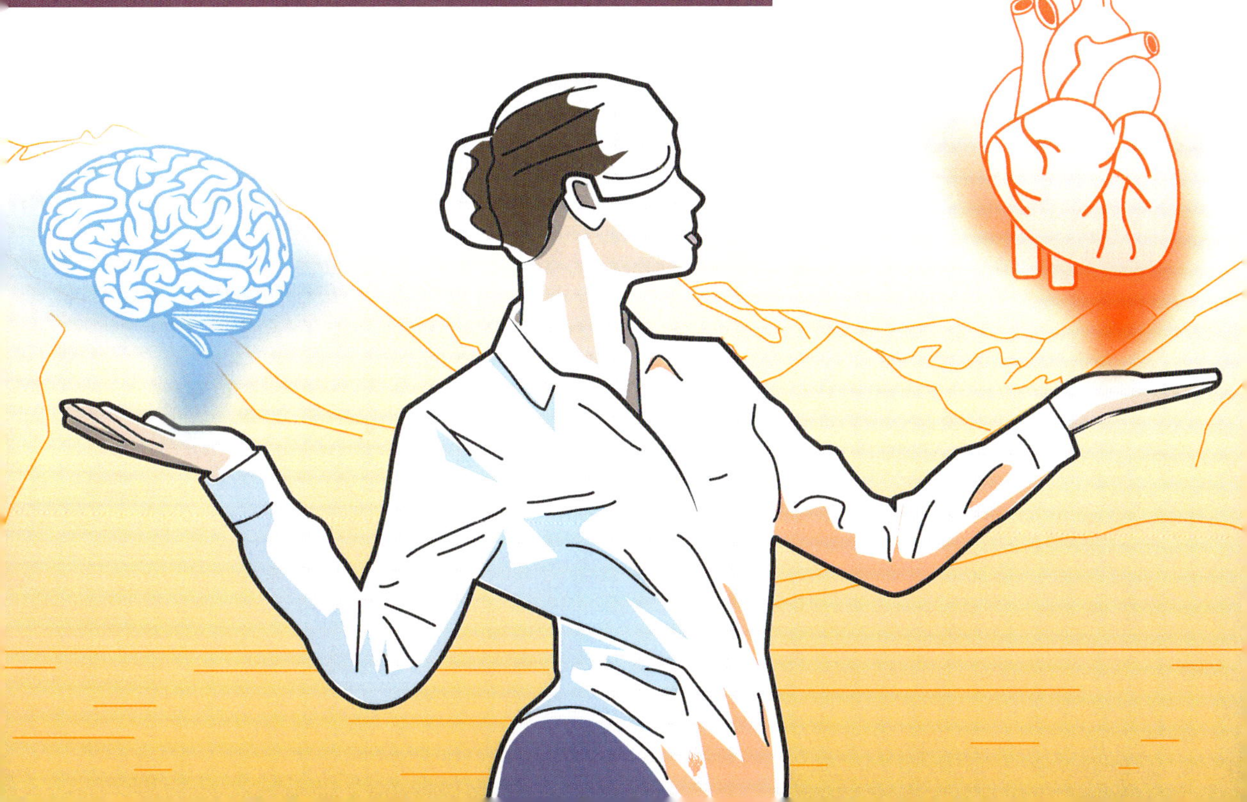

These characters also fall into two main subgroups:

- Reflective–emotional. These are relaxed and very empathetic people. They tend to be very loyal. They talk slowly and use a lot of words that represent emotions. Stress can make them feel insecure, they can be overwhelmed by emotion and find it hard to reason and think, so they need to take their time. They handle conflict and confrontation poorly.
- Active–emotional. These are very sociable people who talk quickly because they are prone to action and experience emotions intensely. Unlike thoughtful, rational people, they do not like to base their purchasing decisions on product data, instead they are guided by the feelings they will experience by buying the item. As with the previous subgroup, they use a lot of words related to emotions, but even more intensely.

Self-awareness is of great help when identifying each person's predominant communication profile and defining traits in order to achieve more effective communication. This will improve the team's communication style.

A good opportunity to practice this skill is during meetings and day-to-day interaction among the team.

We are visual, auditory, or kinaesthetic communicators

Human beings think in a continuous internal dialogue and perceive reality through their senses, which is particularly relevant in the field of neuromarketing because the predominant sensory system differs from one person to another. These systems refer to the way information is collected and interpreted by the mind.

Some people are more likely to communicate using visual language, others prefer auditory information, and some are kinaesthetic.

The mode of communication established will depend on the type of nonverbal communication employed and which sensory channel is used. If managers become skilful detectors and sharpen their perceptive ability, they will be able to tune in to their team's sensory frequencies and therefore understand them better and making themselves better understood.

Visual people think through images, their brains work faster, and they talk quickly and in a high tone.

Auditory people incorporate more information through sound, hence they are active listeners.

Synaesthesia is the joint assimilation or interference of two or more sensory pathways, so people are said to hear colours, see sounds, or associate textures with flavours. Some people are more likely to use synaesthesia than others, for example they may associate wellbeing and serenity with a particular colour, or an aroma with a specific feeling. This phenomenon is culture specific and frequently exploited in neuromarketing.

If you consider different synaesthesias, cultural preferences, the values and beliefs of people working together in a clinic, besides establishing harmony between staff, you could also create a pleasant atmosphere for clients visiting the clinic for the first time.

Identifying a person's most distinctive traits is like having a dictionary to help interpret and select their preferred communication style. It provides the key to being understood by someone who previously spoke in an unknown language.

In neuromarketing, this skill can become so important that it tips the balance between succeeding or failing in a sale, or between the personal satisfaction or dissatisfaction of clients, both internal and external.

Neuromarketing and neurolinguistic programming

Neurolinguistic programming (NLP) is a science that began in the early 1970s, pioneered by John Grinder and Richard Bandler in Santa Cruz, California. As it developed, it soon divided into two perspectives: as a process to discover the patterns and characteristics that people use to excel in a field; and on the other hand, as a technique to observe and analyse the effective means of thinking and communicating of people who excelled at what they did, even if they did not know how they did it.

Neuromarketing and NLP are complementary in that they study how the human mind functions in regard to how we perceive the world through our senses, that is, how the brain organises what we see, hear, and feel, and how this information is filtered and encoded.

Many studies have concluded that eye movements constitute clues as to which part of the brain (hemisphere) is being used, as well as indicating the importance of paying attention to verbal and nonverbal language.

A visual communicator will direct their gaze to the upper right or left sides depending on whether they are remembering or constructing a mental image. Whereas someone who processes information audibly will move their eyes horizontally, because they are constructing a memory based on a sound.

If a person's eyes look downwards, a kinaesthetic process is predominating, that is, they are receiving physical sensations.

EXERCISE

Ask your conversation partner these questions and watch their eye movement.

- WHAT COLOUR ARE YOUR BEDROOM WALLS?
- DO YOU REMEMBER YOUR FAVOURITE SONG?
- HOW DO YOU FEEL WHEN STANDING CLOSE TO A FIREPLACE?

Watching eye movements can help you understand how the other person thinks so you can choose appropriate strategies to improve communication. For example, if you notice someone predominantly uses their visual communication channel, they will appreciate even the most basic diagram. Hence the success of infographics as communication tools.

NLP pays special attention to the words a speaker uses because they define their beliefs and convictions. The choice of words evokes images, sounds, or sensations. Words assume the meaning that they have assigned to them in previous experiences.

Choosing the right words will result in successful communication with your team. Simplifications can distort the message you wish to get across, thus leading to misunderstandings.

Words can also help clarify the objections of the person you are speaking with. One example is the (frequently subconscious) use of the word "but", which is so often used by our internal clients. A "but" invalidates everything that precedes it in a sentence. "I think it is only fair that we share the emergency shifts, but if I could change some of my days off..."

A "but" is often used when someone is not convinced by a suggested solution or proposal. You should take it as an opportunity to find out what is really worrying them.

In conclusion, words are so powerful they can produce a "Pygmalion effect". According to Wikipedia, the expectations a leader places on a follower can influence the follower's performance. In other words, positive, encouraging communication with staff will improve their effectiveness and performance.

Communication and rapport in a job interview

Although the number of veterinary surgeons is increasing worldwide, it is often said that it is hard to find the right staff.

A job interview can be the beginning of a long relationship. Both the interviewer and candidate should prepare for the interview as it is really a form of trade negotiation.

During the interview, everything that is said, how both parties dress and sit, and the para- and metalanguage they use are all processed subconsciously. Akin to a purchasing decision, judgements are made quickly and impulsively using subconscious parameters.

The primitive brain is continuously analysing and evaluating, and the person maintains an internal dialogue which distracts them from active listening.

When candidates are asked what they value in a job their immediate response is usually the timetable (their assessment of the balance between the working hours and amount of time remaining for their personal life), salary (the security provided by a monthly income), and possession of a stable contract (certainty and stability).

When the issue is examined further and other aspects regarding team relationships are explored, many more hidden needs emerge. What feelings and emotions will influence their decision to work for the company? The candidate will consider the stress and fatigue the new job will generate, as well as their motivation. If they have endured a bad experience in another job, their negative memories will affect their future decisions. Their reptilian brain will put them on alert, even though it is a new job with different conditions. It is amazing how all this can occur subconsciously and in the blink of an eye during an interview.

Job interview

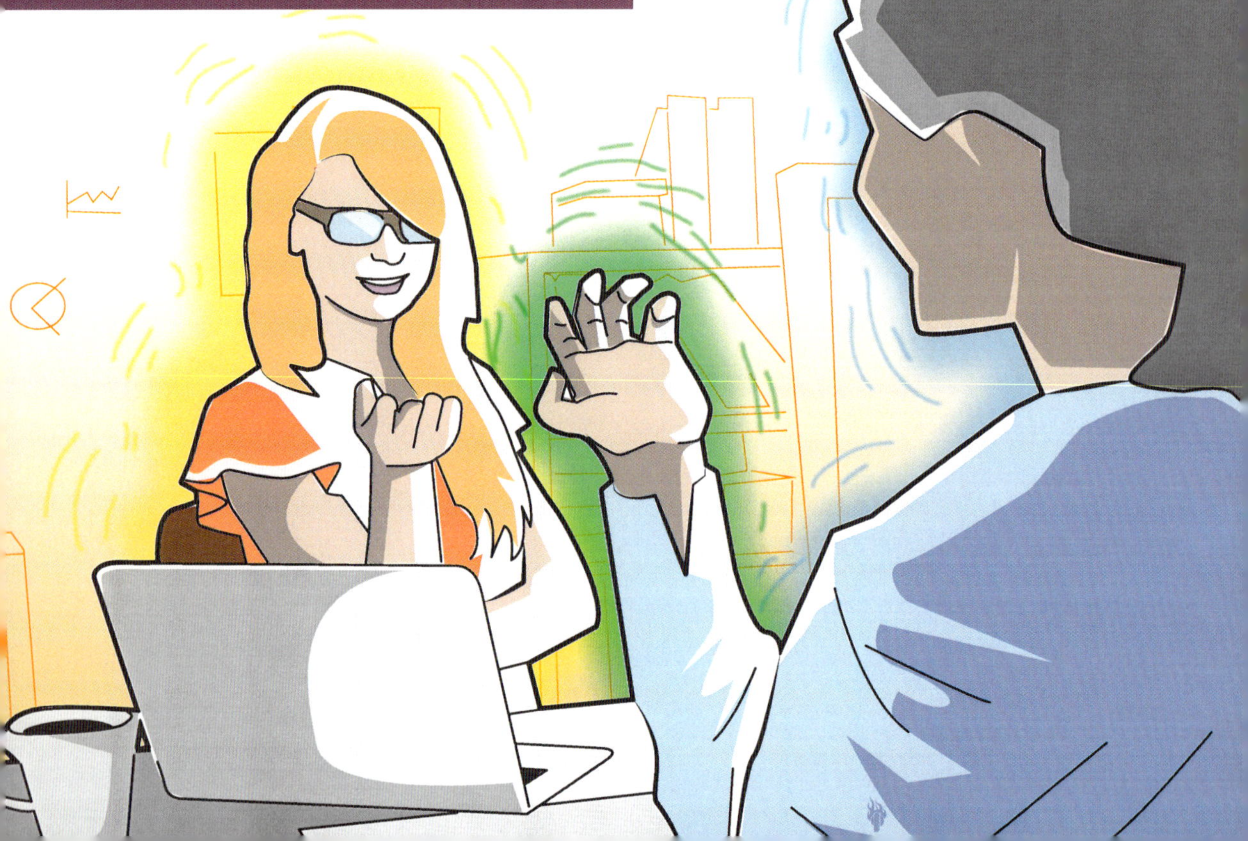

By contrast, the interviewer may have an urgent need to fill a vacancy (e.g. due to an unexpected period of sick leave) and therefore conduct a less stringent interview. However, if they are recruiting for a position in a new service or speciality, they will take more time and place the utmost emphasis on the quality of the candidate.

Posture is also very important during a job interview. A strong rapport can help form a connection and instil confidence, which can be transmitted to the other person through empathy, thus creating harmony and improving communication. When a good rapport is established, people's gestures, tone of voice, and oral fluency all synchronise.

When two people are in tune, their bodies adopt the same posture, they subconsciously imitate the way the other person crosses their legs, or moves their arms, head, or hands. Sometimes their breathing also harmonises.

Efficient meetings to improve the implementation of processes

Efficient meetings are held regularly, but without going beyond the time that is strictly necessary. Their quality does not particularly depend on how long they last, but on how information is organised, moderated, and managed, and whether all participants can agree on conclusions, assuming responsibilities, and committing to an ongoing assessment of what they have decided to put it into practice.

In meetings, everyone should feel they can contribute their ideas and the needs of each team member must be considered when undertaking sales and/or marketing projects.

The manager or head of the meeting will be responsible for resolving issues in the best and quickest manner possible.

Factors that can benefit meetings

All attendees should try to participate in the meeting. There are always time-thieves and people who do not let others speak. As explained earlier, people with an active personality will give their opinion more readily than reflective people.

Everyone should be encouraged to give their opinion, including those who are reluctant to speak because they are shy or only joined the company recently. There are tools to help these people get heard, such as brainwriting (see next page for an example).

A PRACTICAL EXAMPLE OF BRAINWRITING

The purpose of this exercise is to focus a meeting on a subject you believe will be good for your clinic's positioning:

- Organise a meeting with your team to find out what differentiates your company from the competition.
- It may surprise you that the answer is not always clear; they may also be aware of the differences, but they may not have fully absorbed them or be unsure how to communicate them to the end client.
- The meeting will verify whether the management and internal clients share the same ideas regarding the company's strengths or, on the contrary, it may give light to a new vision for creating a new strategic plan.
- The ability to communicate with and understand clients (internal and external) will help differentiate your company from others and encourage them to purchase your services and products.

Staff sense of belonging and social acceptance in your clinic

Social acceptance consists of forming part of a group, whether friends, a sports team, or a work team. The person identifies with the rest of the members with whom they share, either consciously or subconsciously, the same values and habits.

This sense of belonging is heavily exploited by brands. An obvious example is that of a football club, wherein the supporters regard the successes and failures of their team as their own and the results even affect their mood. A sense of belonging produces wellbeing among the group, they complete tasks more successfully, and it improves the company's goals and profitability.

What happens when the bond between the company and its employees breaks down? What happens between workmates?

This gives rise to an unwanted situation where rivalry, leadership battles, and whispers in the corridor increase and result in conflicts; employees criticise their bosses and coworkers, and the team is split into two groups: those "for" and "against".

Can I stimulate and influence a sense of belonging?

Individual recognition, a certain degree of independence, and freedom of choice are important factors when trying to make people feel part of a team.

The leader must know how to convey to the team that each member is important because they know the clients, their pets and their needs, the suppliers and sales reps.

They must encourage two-way communication whereby everyone feels motivated, involved with the company's values, and able to participate by offering ideas and opinions.

You can create an emotional link by organising company meals to celebrate important dates, giving small gifts on birthdays, or celebrating important life events such as weddings, births, or the adoption of a child.

Although it is hard to achieve, you will know that you have done it when you notice that employees are happy and want to continue working at your clinic.

Employees as internal clients

"I once attended a course with a veterinary assistant who owned three dogs. During the conversation he mentioned he did not buy dog food at the clinic because we only sold expensive brands and it would cost him too much since he had three dogs, so he bought their food at the supermarket."

This is a clear example of a failure to gain the loyalty of an internal client and therefore it will be hard to earn the loyalty of the clinic's end clients.

If your company has a staff discount policy in place, the prices must be explicitly defined. Discounts help sell products, which ensures your staff, or salespeople, are familiar with the items they are selling. If they become consumers, they can spread both product information as well as their emotional experience.

Your discount policy must be in writing, and uniform and standardised for all employees. If possible, add it to the management programme, so discounts are carried out directly, which is simple when they are applied as a percentage of the product or service.

Important factors to consider when writing your discounts policy

- Use straightforward, understandable language which leaves no room for misunderstandings.
- All employees must be familiar with the document.
- Give a copy to everyone in the team and retain one copy in the clinic.
- Apply different types of discount based on the groups of services and products: food, parasite treatments, vaccinations, appointments, surgery, etc.
- Specify who exactly can receive the employee discounts; you must state in writing whether each discount is also applicable to relatives or friends.
- Discounts will only be applicable so long as the payment is made within the established period.
- You should state that the discount policy will be periodically reviewed, for example, once a year.
- The company reserves the right to create, modify, or withdraw any of the discounts.

- Additionally, you could offer staff commissions or incentives linked to sales volumes, depending on whether the product is part of a campaign, offer, or promotion. The commission could be customised to each employee according to their position and duties.
- Include the loyalty cards offered by laboratories or pet food suppliers; for example, discounts for volumes purchased over a specific period.
- Employees should perceive the discounts as recognition and reward for their work at the company.
- Discounts that may be applied to the end client. You should include clients who have products such as health plans which make them eligible for discounts, which must also be standardised and reported to all staff.

Company stakeholders are also clients

The company must cover the expectations and needs of all stakeholders. An agreement between stakeholders is a written document that reinforces commercial trust and stability.

Each time you suggest purchasing a new piece of diagnostic equipment, developing a new campaign, defining your employees' incentives, and even their salaries, there is a round of negotiation followed by a sales process.

Your partners are also clients and you must have mutual trust, share a single company mission and vision, and agree on strategic decisions.

The owner is responsible for earning the team's loyalty

The clinic's owner or manager must ensure that staff know their duties and provide a good service. They must also be a happiness manager, in other words, a leader who generates harmony and moments of delight, and is able to meet the needs of their internal clients.

EXAMPLE

You are divorced and, since you spend so many hours at work, your ex-partner calls the clinic to ask you to collect the children from school this afternoon because he or she will be late. You get angry because you are also working, and you recall raw emotions from when you were fighting for custody, which translate into feelings and thoughts of increasing discomfort. Eventually you agree and will rearrange your schedule since you are the boss. You call your employee vet who had the afternoon off and tell them they must cover your shift because you have a family problem. As you are already in a bad mood, you speak in a commanding tone. Your vet comes into the clinic. However, what you do not realise is that they had to ring their ex-partner to ask them to collect the children and they are very angry with you and your company.

Your mission as a manager is to retain your employees, as you have invested time in interviews, training, and harmonising the team. This effort should translate into loyalty towards your company. If your employees are committed, they will help build client loyalty.

The famous comfort zone

Another hidden staff requirement is the need to feel secure, to remain within a stable entity. Companies need flexible workers who can adapt to changes. However, if the basic salary portion of their overall income does not cover their rent or mortgage, petrol, food, monthly bills, and a long list of other family living costs, will they be motivated by incentives and commissions or will they suffer a monthly bout of anxiety and stress? Incentives can be double-edged swords; they must be managed correctly to satisfy the motivation they can generate.

The possession of an internal company policy manual, which you should review annually with your staff and update if necessary, would also impart confidence. Ultimately, this agreement is a contract with your team that is built on mutual trust between both parties.

Are you a leader for your internal clients?

In their book *A Passion for Excellence* (1983), Tom Peters and Nancy Austin offer a relatively comprehensive description of what leadership should be:

"Leadership means vision, cheerleading, enthusiasm, love, trust, verve, passion, obsession, consistency, the use of symbols, paying attention (...), coaching, effectively wandering around, and numerous other things. Leadership must be present at all levels of the organisation. It depends on a million little things done with obsession, consistency and care, but all of those million little things add up to nothing if the trust, vision and basic belief are not there."

T. Peters and N. Austin, A Passion for Excellence: The Leadership Difference

The owner or manager of a company must know how to differentiate whether they are fulfilling the role of a manager or that of a leader.

The latter goes beyond the role of a manager; without detriment to the difficulty and importance of being an excellent manager, an excellent leader must have foresight and the ability to explore the full potential of their veterinary practice.

Another difference is that a leader must be able to define the goals and results they wish to achieve, using their ability to motivate and inspire their employees by making them feel like key parts of the engine that moves the organisation, whereas a manager's duties are limited to planning and supervising.

Transforming yourself into a good leader implies learning how to incite action, based on the conviction that what really matters in a company are the people. The belief that a team need only carry out their contacted duties, without motivating the members to express and develop their creative ideas, opinions, and inspirations, is a concept held by a manager.

A leader must allow their team to get involved beyond their assigned duties and commit themselves to the clinic's common goals by encouraging individual initiatives.

The organisation must have information about the company's fluctuations, any changes in stakeholders and legal situations, available resources, and the requirements and expectations they must fulfil to continue performing optimally. They should also receive feedback about the results obtained as a team.

A good leader must provide support and resolve the team's needs so that it may carry out projects efficiently and pleasantly. For example, they need to keep abreast of whether employees have a space to work and drink a coffee, if computers are up-to-date, if equipment used to treat wounds, perform diagnostic tests or operations, etc., is adequate and in good condition. All this creates an atmosphere of confidence and security in which the team opts to take risks and get actively and enthusiastically involved, which translates into good results and profits for the company as everyone wins and nobody loses.

If things do not initially work out this way, maybe it is because you find it hard to stop acting like a manager. To make the change you only need motivation, commitment, and self-criticism, or the ability to observe other companies that could serve as a model, or you could even get help from a coach.

The team and your clients: a systemic vision

The perception clients have of your company's cohesion and good atmosphere accounts for 50 % of your clinic's success, taking on even greater importance than the quality of your products and services. Everything perceived as positive or negative (e.g. leaders and the team) will have an influence on clients.

If we imagine three people throwing stones into a lake at the same time and close together, they will create ripples that eventually merge together and therefore each has an influence on the others. As soon as the stones fall into the water they become interrelated and interconnected. This is parallel to the concept of organisational systems within companies.

Transferring this example to your team, you might think that any change, decision, or operation you undertake will trigger an effect that influences each team member. Therefore, if you provoke unhappiness in one employee (e.g. through unfair treatment, passiveness when opposing subgroups emerge, incentives based solely on production and without considering each individual's value and respect, etc.), the ripples will inevitably expand until they finally reach your external clients.

Companies are systems composed of subsystems, such as the veterinary team and the auxiliary personnel. Both subsystems are interrelated and strive for a common objective. What is more, everyone has their own systems, including their partner, family, and friends, who also affect them and will influence in decisions relative to the company, for example, changes in their working hours and vacations.

Since these subsystems are interdependent, any change in one of them will affect the others and have positive or negative consequences for the company's profitability.

The team will not function as a collective if each member has different goals because their individual objectives may not be aligned to, or may even contradict, the company's overall objectives.

In summary, to start adopting a systemic vision of the company and its work teams, you must become familiar with five key points.

A system is said to be in synergy when the teams work together, combining their potential as individuals and attaining the desired goal more quickly and efficiently.

Work teams

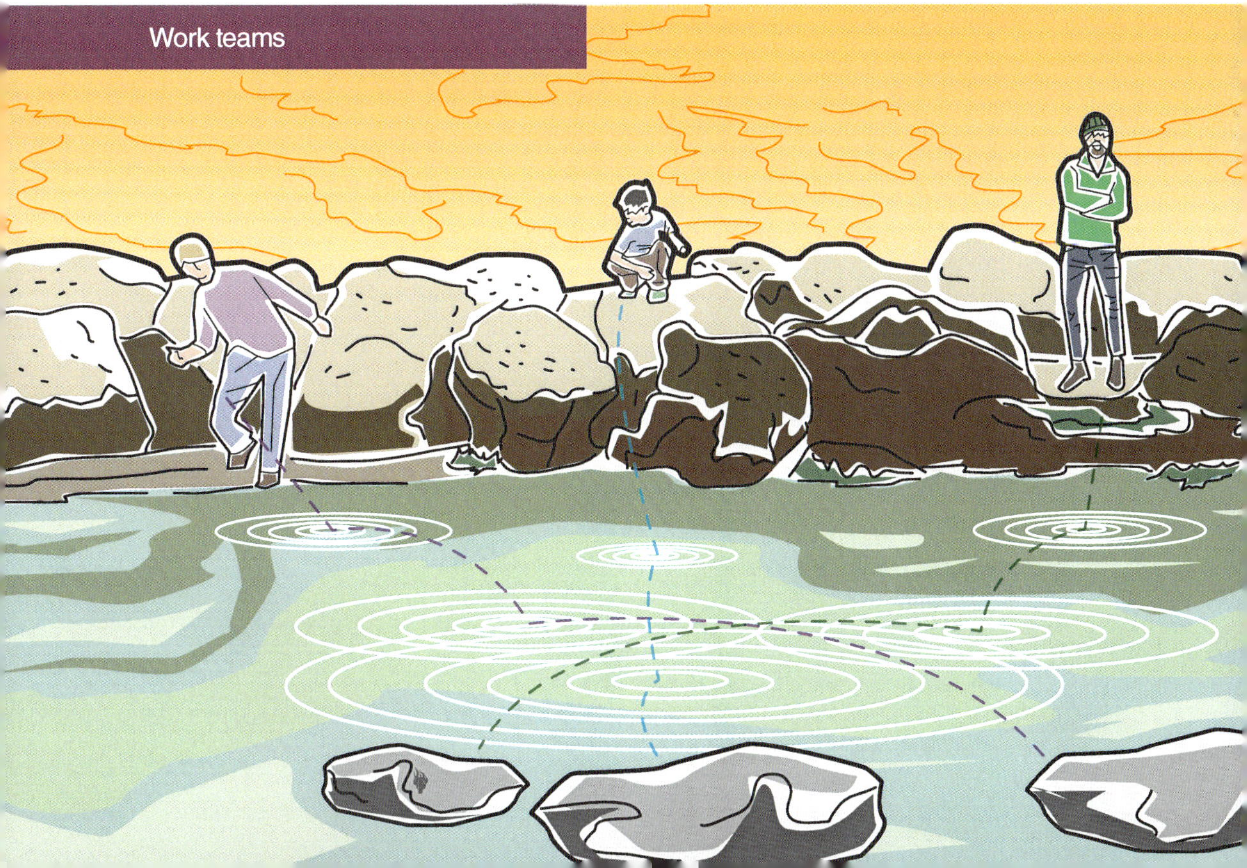

5 KEY POINTS

1. People are not isolated entities, they are always interrelated with others.
2. People lose their individual role to form part of the system or company. When searching for individual solutions, they offer short-term benefits, whereas global solutions present long-term benefits.
3. Modification or change in each member has a knock-on effect on the whole team.
4. People not only belong to a single system; their internal situation influences their needs and decisions.
5. Goals are achieved with less effort when working in a team.

When one team member vibrates at a different frequency from the rest, the system develops inefficiencies, it starts to degrade and break down, thereby disrupting communication and collaboration between employees. Consequently, this will have a negative impact on your company's economic results and the team's motivation.

Conclusions

Familiarity with your internal clients will reduce the number of conflicts, increase confidence within the team, induce motivation, improve involvement in the creation, dissemination, and advertising of campaigns, health plans, and sales, and enrich the quality of relationships. This will result in a pleasant working atmosphere and foster the feeling of belonging within the team.

The sum of all these factors will mark the difference for your company, not necessarily contributing to the points which make you better than other companies, but instead emphasising the qualities that make your clinic stand out from the rest, thus reducing the number of clients who abandon your clinic and increasing profitability and efficiency, both internally and externally.

17 Tools for implementing neuromarketing in a veterinary practice

Before developing your neuromarketing plan and implementing any new procedures, it is important to ensure the changes you make are aligned to your company's mission, vision, and corporate values, as explained in Chapter 5. You should put your plan in writing, include systematic and structured content, and clearly identify who is responsible for each procedure. Impatience and immediacy can lead to decisions that seem like good ideas at first, but which later stray from the plan. But there is no need to worry; in this chapter we present some templates that will help you draft and implement your clinic's neuromarketing plan.

Obviously, the ultimate goal is to boost your number of clients, increase your average transaction, reinforce client loyalty, recover clients who abandon your centre, develop a good policy for capturing new clients, and, above all, increase the clinic's profitability.

Alfred Hitchcock once said, "To make a great film you need three things – the script, the script, and the script."

Firstly, we suggest you dedicate some time to drawing up a good plan and deciding on what you will do, how, and when.

In our sector, losses endured due to the rise of new sales channels or legislative changes force us to concentrate on furnishing our veterinary services with added value. In some countries, this is coupled with a wide array of professionals in a market that cannot absorb them all, but who set up new clinics and therefore generate intense competitive pressure and cheap opportunities for pet owners to change clinics.

We have already mentioned that veterinary services are intangible and consumed immediately, that is why factors such as the impression you cause, your friendliness, behaviour, your practice's location or nearby parking facilities will influence the client's purchasing experience. This intangibility means consumers may perceive a difference between the veterinary service offered by different clinics, and this is what neuromarketing aims to achieve.

Diagnosing your initial situation

You must know how to analyse your baseline situation. To this end, you can employ the tools explained hereafter.

SWOT analysis

SWOT is an acronym for strengths, weaknesses, opportunities, and threats.

- Weaknesses: the company's internal weak points that harm your ability to meet your goals.
- Strengths: the company's strong points that increase your chances of meeting your objectives.
- Threats: factors outside the company that could impair your clinic from fulfilling its established goals and objectives.
- Opportunities: elements outside the company that could be employed to help the business achieve its proposed goals and objectives.

Table 1. SWOT analysis.

Weaknesses	Threats
■ My practice does not have any scent or fragrance. ■ I cannot always answer the phone in reception.	A new clinic with expertise in neuromarketing is about to open.
Strengths	**Opportunities**
My client database is very well segmented.	The local council has decided to install a dog toilet area close to my veterinary practice.

CAME analysis

Based on the SWOT analysis (Table 1), you can create a CAME (correct, adapt, maintain, explore) table (Table 2) to identify the basic actions available.

Table 2. CAME analysis.

Correct	Adapt
How can I correct the weaknesses noted in the SWOT analysis? Actions I could implement.	What actions could I implement to address the threats in the SWOT analysis?
Maintain	**Explore**
Actions to continue developing my strengths.	How can I react to new opportunities? Actions I could implement.

Select the points from the CAME table that fulfil the following requisites:

1. Select the action that reaches the most or most desirable clients. Remember the Pareto principle states that 80 % of your revenue will come from 20–30 % of your clients. The action you choose must have the largest or most immediate effect; maintain your clients segmented in accordance with the Pareto principle.
2. The effort required to develop it must not hamper you from developing other projects you have selected. Your initial choices should be the easiest to implement.
3. You have sufficient resources to carry out the selected actions.

This will give you a snapshot of your current position and what you can do to develop the desired strategy in a certain period. You should avoid trying to take on all the actions at the same time; attempting to resolve all the points may lead to failure and, in turn, frustration and demotivation.

Analysing the competition

Comparison table

Before going any further, we recommend you analyse your competitors and compare your situation against theirs in a neuromarketing context (Table 3).

Table 3. Analysis of the competition.

Feature under comparison	"The Laurels" clinic, my practice	"CanDog" hospital	"4 paws" clinic
Opening hours	Normal business hours	24 hours	Normal business hours
Emergencies	Agreement with a third party; home ambulance service	Yes	No
Up-to-date website	Yes	Unchanged for quite some time	No website
Social media	Yes	Yes	Extensive use of SM, particularly Facebook
Piped music	No	No	Yes
Scented rooms	Yes	Yes	No
Centre-coherent uniforms	Yes	No	Yes
Fulfils the principle of coherence	Yes	No	Yes
Pet grooming service	Yes	No	Yes
Appointment requests via WhatsApp	Yes	No	Yes
Appointment requests via Facebook	Yes	No	Yes
Offers health plans	Yes	No	No
Location	Town centre	Outskirts	Neighbourhood
Parking	Yes, town centre parking	Private parking	No

Mind map

A mind map (Fig. 1) is a diagram used to help organise information. It provides an outline of the key points in each implementation phase and the actions to carry out in a given period.

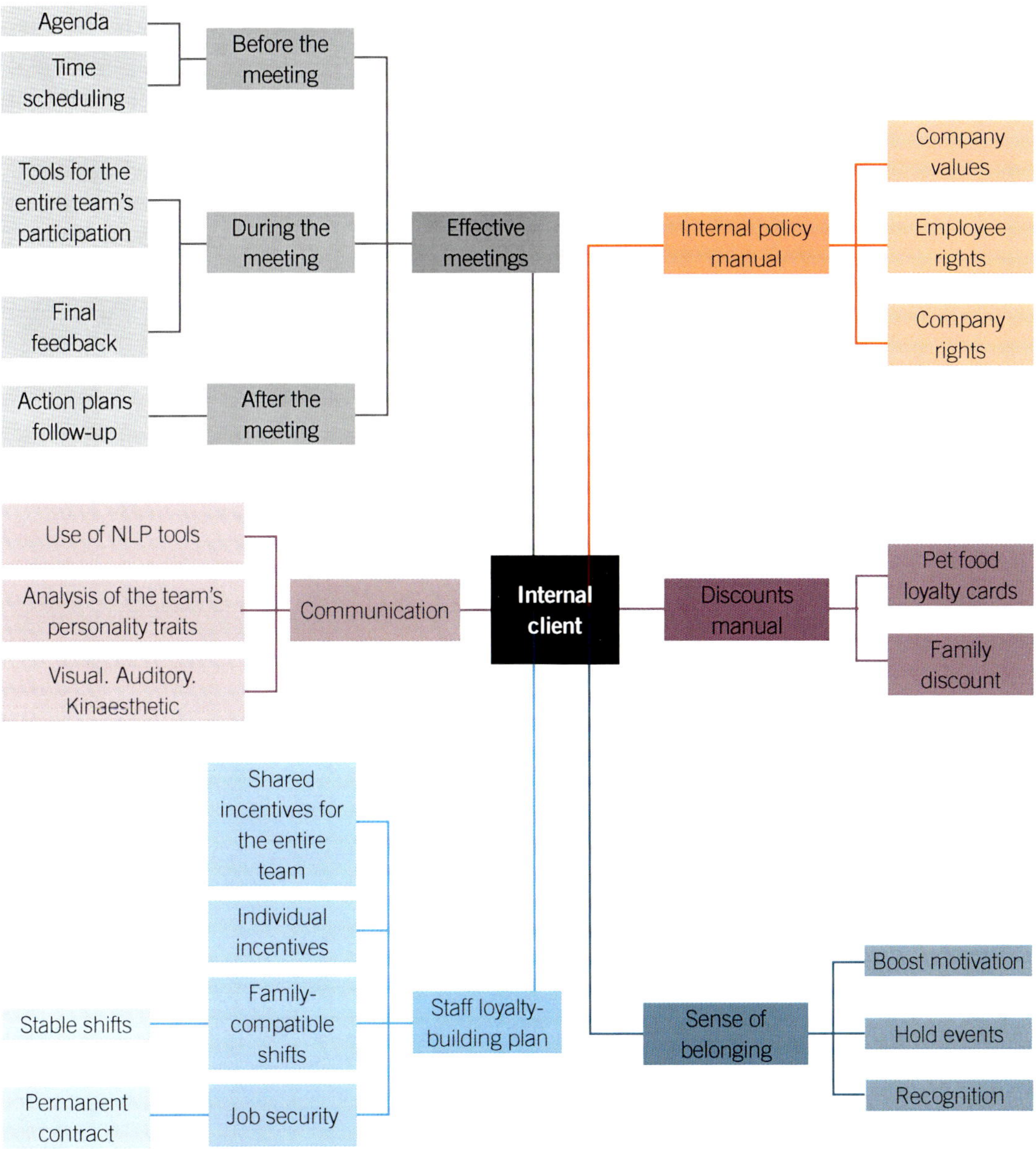

Figure 1. Example of a mind map.

Ishikawa diagram

Ishikawa diagrams, also called fishbone diagrams, are used to perform a thorough analysis of each aspect associated with a specific problem (Fig. 2).

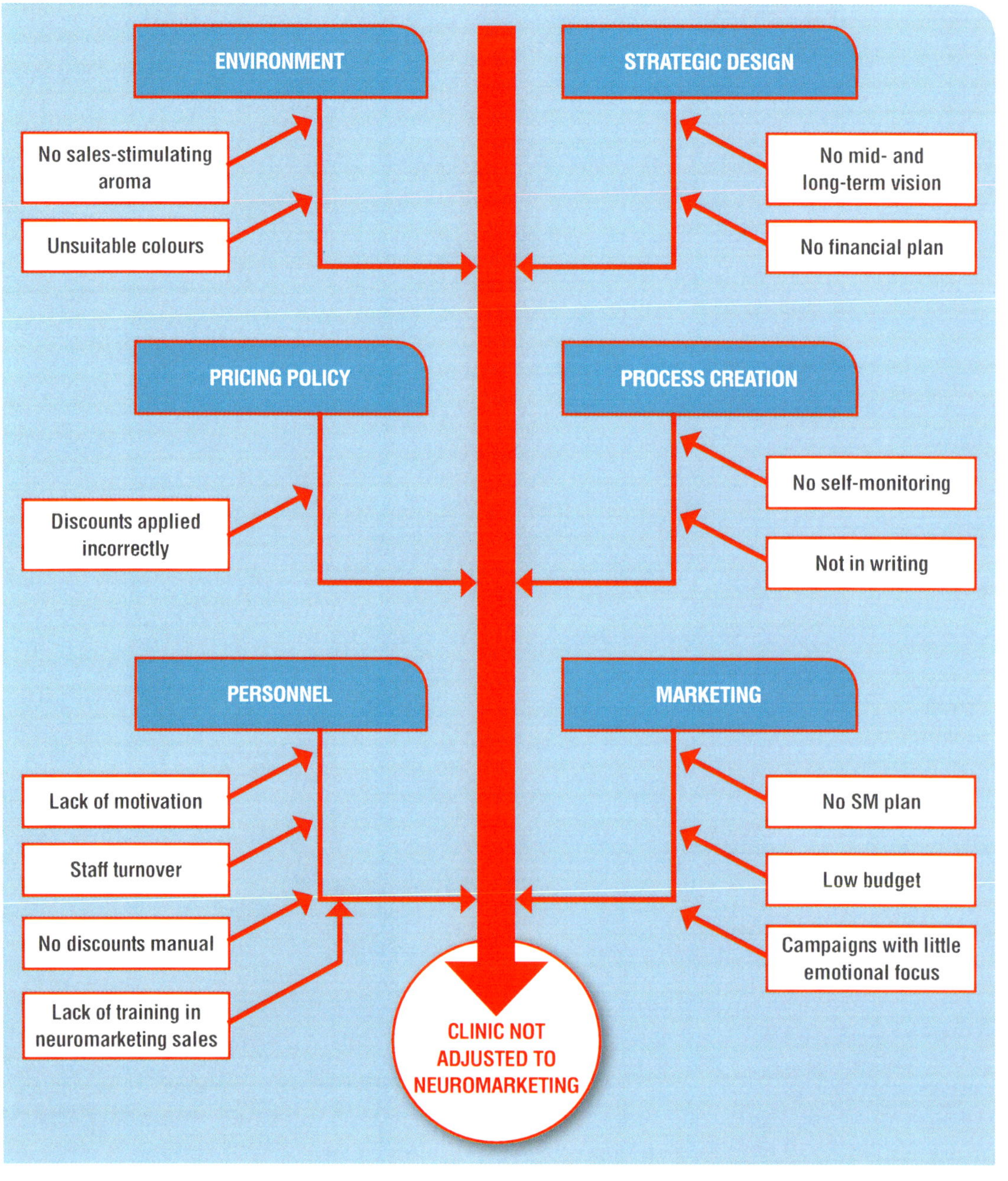

Figure 2. Example of an Ishikawa diagram.

Client analysis

Segmentation

Steps for defining your client

Demographic data

Extract demographic data about your town from official data held by local councils or your country's national institute of statistics. You can classify the population by neighbourhoods, age groups, sex, socioeconomic level.

Define your client's profile

You must analyse what your clients are like; what needs do they have? You must therefore count on a good CRM system to help segment your data correctly. The final objective is to identify your ideal client, so you may create value propositions which earn their loyalty. An attractive suggestion is put forward in the book *Value Proposition Design* by Osterwalder et al, where he develops a tool which firstly works on your client's profile before creating a value map for this client.

Client needs

The client visits your clinic in search of solutions. You can define different categories of client needs:

- Functional: food for pets, cleaning products, accessories for going for walks, substrates for exotic pets.
- Veterinary: disease prevention, vaccinations, and deworming and flea and tick control treatments.
- Social: clients can join clubs for agility training, puppies, different breeds, etc. Belonging to a group is one of our basic human needs, as discussed earlier.
- Emotional: clients love their pets and in return they receive affection, company, or security. They often tell us about their animals' feelings.

One recommendation is to elaborate a list of your current clients' needs. To discover these needs, you can ask yourself the following questions:

- Why do they visit your practice?
- Why do people go to other clinics? What do they offer which you don't?
- What are their concerns about their pets?
- What is their level of knowledge about a recently acquired pet?
- Do most of your clients adopt pets or do they purchase them?
- Is their animal just a pet or is it also a working animal?

As a manager, there are a lot more questions you could ask until you have defined the profile of the ideal client to whom you will offer different value propositions.

You can also create another classification of client needs by dividing them into two groups. This division depends on the following:

- Expressed needs: these are normally linked to their basic and expected needs.
- Latent needs: these are more to do with desired and unexpected needs (necessities the salesperson can perceive, needs that neither the client nor the salesperson is consciously aware of).

The following figure describes another method for classifying client needs (Fig. 3).

CLASSIFICATION OF CLIENT NEEDS

1. *Basic needs available at your practice:*
   food, complementary items.
2. *Expected needs:*
   vaccinations, parasite control products, veterinary services.
3. *Desirable needs:*
   long opening hours and emergency services.
4. *Unexpected needs:*
   to go beyond the client's expectations. They are unaware you have, for example, your own laboratory or training courses.

DEWORMING TREATMENT ADMINISTERED AS IF IT WERE A TREAT. THIS CREATES A GAME WITH THE CLIENT'S PET

EASY TO PURCHASE (ONLINE VERSUS PHYSICAL ATTENTION)

THE CLIENT NEEDS TO DEWORM THEIR PET

Figure 3. Classification of client needs.

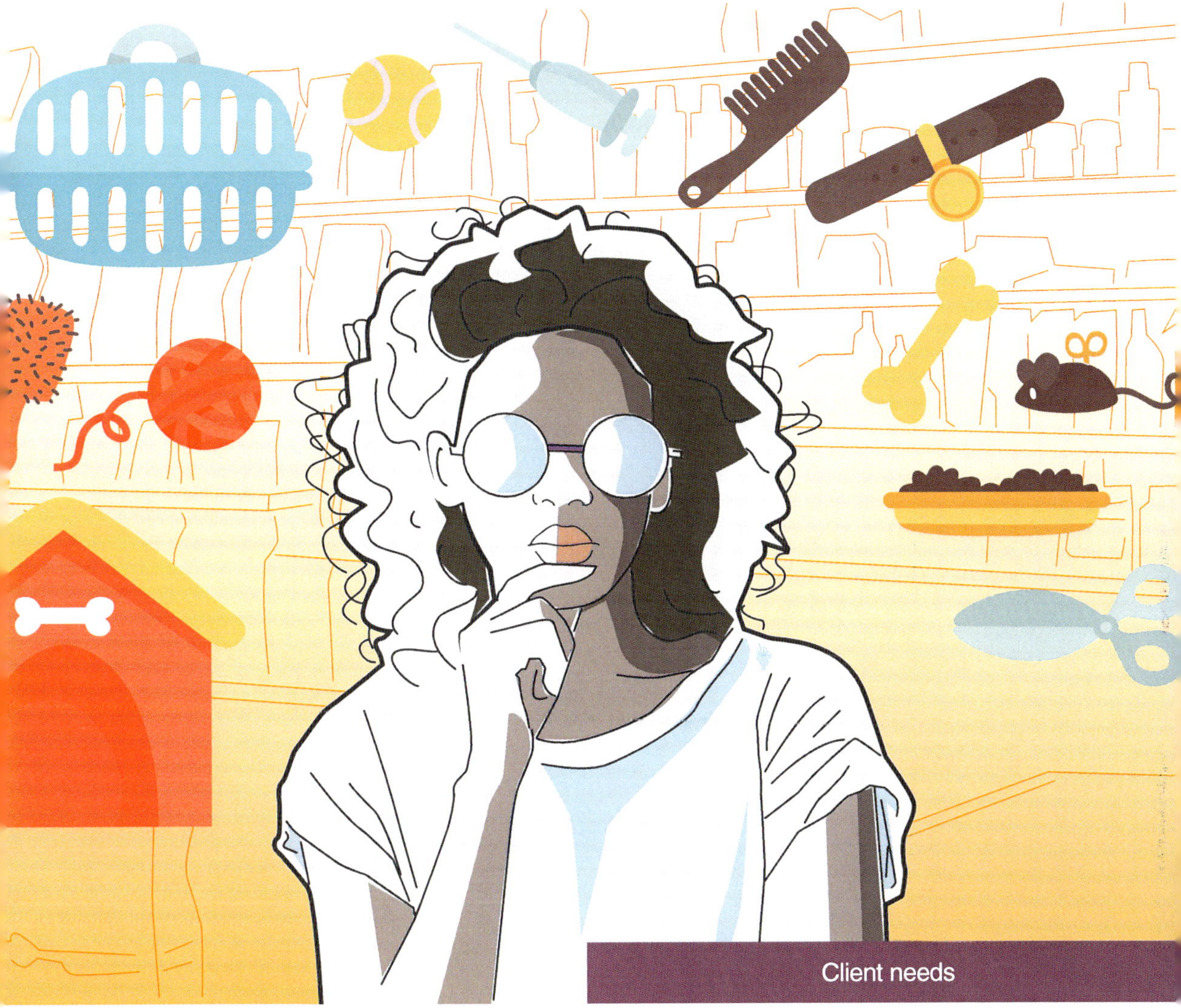

It is vitally important that the value proposition is adapted to the client's needs because it will affect how they perceive the quality of the service. If the perceived quality is high, there is a greater chance they will recommend your clinic to potential clients, both online and offline.

To discover if you are on the right track, you can also apply the "Johari window", a technique created in 1955 by the psychologists Joseph Luft and Harry Ingham, to whom it owes its name. Applied to neuromarketing, it serves to identify your relationship with your clients and your knowledge of their needs (Fig. 4).

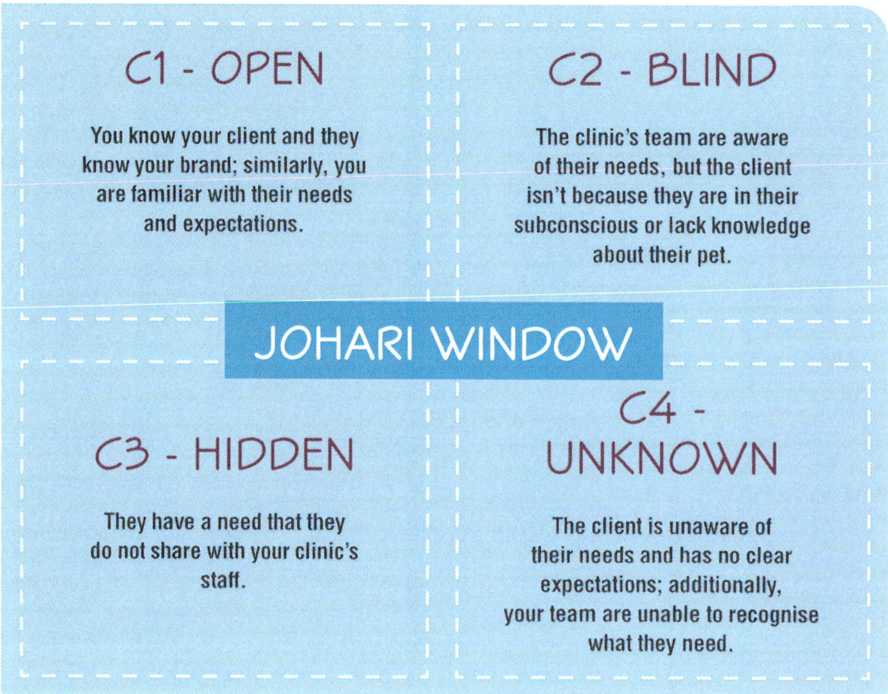

Figure 4. Johari window.

Factors contributing to the client's experience

Strategic experiential modules

The client's experience is influenced by several factors. The aim is to generate positive emotions to minimise negative ones, thus earning greater loyalty and more recommendations for your veterinary centre. Here we present a tool designed by Bernd H. Schmitt which divides client experiences into five generic types known as strategic experiential modules, or SEM (Fig. 5). This classification makes it easier to work on the behaviour patterns of the clients you wish to target.

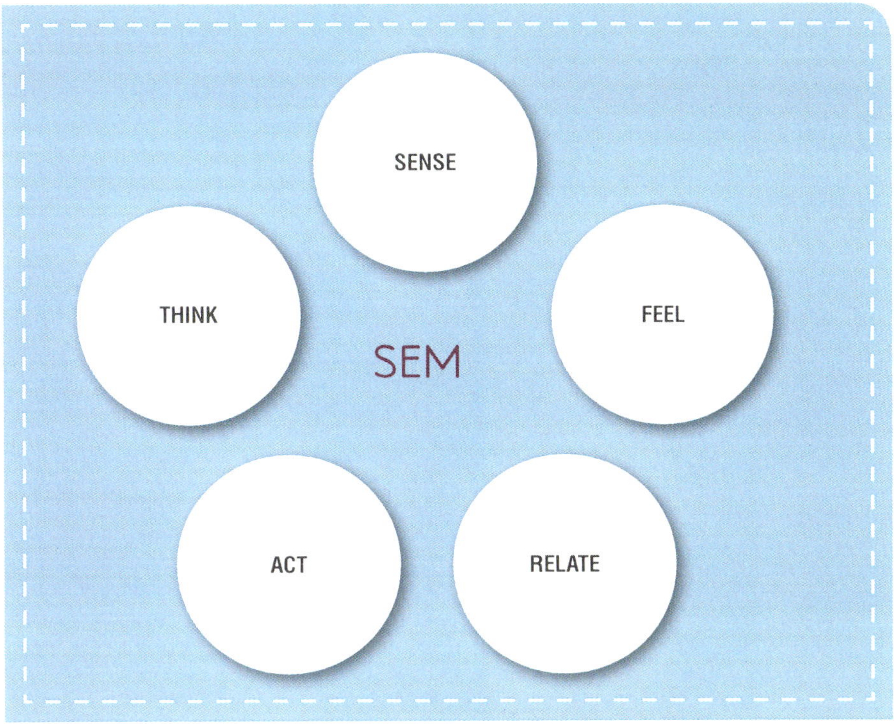

Figure 5. Strategic experiential modules (SEM).

Client life cycle (customer journey)

These are the stages and states a client goes through when interacting with your veterinary practice, regardless of their pet's age. They should not be confused with patient stages (from puppy to elderly dog), as a new client could enter the clinic with a senior pet.

The client cycle considers their motivations and goals, so they always remain loyal to your clinic (Table 4). This cycle must also incorporate the touchpoints (TPs).

Table 4. Strategic experiential modules.

SEM: strategic experiential modules	
Sense	Sensory stimuli perceived through the five primary senses (sight, taste, touch, hearing, and smell). This is where sensory marketing comes into play.
Feel	Appeals to the emotions processed by the brain (joy, empathy, sadness, etc.).
Think	This refers to the mental processes based on the client's creativity with respect to solving problems. They could be convergent (there is only one solution and the client reaches a conclusion) or divergent (there is more than one solution or perspective and the client actively participates in decision-making, thus creating an experience). This module is used extensively in the technology sector.
Act	Physical experiences. Behaviours or lifestyle. For instance, "Coca Cola" makes you smile (happiness).
Relate	This is linked to the other four generic experiences. The experience should have a positive influence in a social context and the desire to be recognised in this context. This is where the desire to belong comes into play, for example, a club card.

Definition of emotion: a neutral, negative, or positive state that we experience because of an action performed to fulfil a need*.

You must bear in mind that retention is increasingly difficult because today's client is multitasking; they may enter to buy a parasite treatment and, while waiting to be attended, they could use their mobile phone to buy pet food from an online shop. There are also "superinformed" clients who have all the data on the item they wish to buy.

There are different types of client and, by the same token, they can have different life cycles. You must therefore prioritise the segments that satisfy the Pareto principle (the 80/20 rule), as more segmentation is harder to manage.

EXERCISE

Identify the client needs and expectations during each stage. You need to fill out each box then create the corresponding TPs (Table 5).

*Carver and Scheier, in *Oxford Handbook of Human Action*.

Table 5. Client needs and expectations.

How can they discover you?	First contact or interest in your service	Purchase	Active client. Repeat purchase	Client who has a positive experience, builds loyalty	Recommendation or loss of client
Contact channels are easily found on your website.	Welcome and actively listen to their needs.	Cat beds. Diets for dogs with food allergies.	Flea and tick collars, pipettes, vaccinations, on a regular basis.	You resolve their telephone queries.	They are satisfied clients and would recommend you. Or they do not return.

Touchpoints (TPs) tool

Touchpoints are the moments when the client interacts with the company and forms an impression or emits a judgement, either consciously or subconsciously. They can both tangible and intangible. Some examples include their first impression of your website, the scent upon entering your centre, the staff's uniforms (if they are stained or clean, wrinkled or ironed), greeting and farewells, etc. (Table 6).

All TPs should have a positive effect on the client, although they will only result in an acceptable experience for some clients. As your resources are limited, you must prioritise the creation of experiences at the most critical points or those with the greatest impact, while acceptable encounters will have to suffice for the other points.

TPs can be divided into three stages:

1. Before the purchase
   - Offers.
   - Website.
   - Social media.
2. During the purchase
   - Veterinary care.
   - Attention in reception.
   - Waiting room period.
3. After the purchase
   - Newsletters.
   - Loyalty programmes.
   - Questionnaires or client announcements.

EXERCISE

We suggest you identify the TPs of your business. Remember many are easy to detect, whereas others are much subtler, but no less important. Try to choose the TPs that could have the greatest impact for your client. They are not the same for all clients, which is why good segmentation is so important.

Table 6. Analysis of a clinic's touchpoints.

TP	What experience does it create?	How can this experience be improved?	How can this be implemented?	When can this be implemented?	People responsible for each TP	How will you measure the success of the TP?
■ Website ■ Social media ■ Shopfront						
■ Website contact form ■ Phone call ■ Welcome to the centre						
Buying a loyalty plan						
At least one purchase per month (food, parasite control product, etc.)						
■ Renewing a health plan ■ In the case of a complaint, ensure the client feels very well attended ■ Payment time ■ Saying goodbye						
■ Recommendation to a friend ■ Recommendation in a park (word-of-mouth publicity)						

After preparing a list of touchpoints, introduce the following lines:

- Importance for the client.
- Importance for the veterinary practice.

Resources are generally allocated to improving the client experience.

Positive emotional balance

There are several ratios which have proven valid in terms of a positive emotional experience compared to a negative one. These ratios are:

1. For a good client experience: 5:1 ratio.

1	2	3	4	5	1
POSITIVE EMOTION					NEGATIVE EMOTION

2. How do I counteract a bad client experience?
   - You must create at least three positive emotions (Fig. 6).

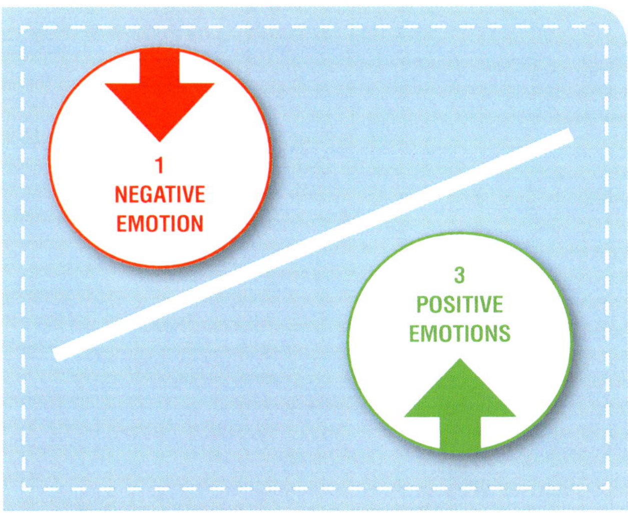

Figure 6. Balance of emotions.
One negative emotion for every three positive emotions.

Philip Kotler defines client satisfaction as "a person's feelings of pleasure or disappointment resulting from comparing a product's perceived performance (or outcome) in relation to his or her expectations".

You should always assess the TPs when defining your targets and action plans, and consider any bad experiences that could occur, as well as the preventive measures to implement to avoid such circumstances arising.

Client satisfaction levels

Client satisfaction after using your services or buying your products can be classified into one of three categories.

1. Dissatisfaction: the service or product did not meet their expectations.
2. Satisfaction: the product or service fulfilled the client's expectations.
3. Gratification: when their expectations are exceeded.

This gives us the equation:

LEVEL OF SATISFACTION = PERCEIVED PERFORMANCE - CLIENT EXPECTATIONS

Considering that:

Perceived performance	
Excellent	10
Good	7
Regular	5
Poor	3

Level of client expectation	
High	3
Moderate	2
Low	1

Level of satisfaction			
Exceeds expectations	Positive satisfaction	8 to 10	Excellent service
Meets expectations	Neutral satisfaction	5 to 7	Acceptable, appropriate service
Does not meet expectations	Dissatisfaction	≤4	Poor, inadequate, and deficient service

If a satisfaction survey yielded results indicating the perceived performance was good, equal to a score of 7, but expectations were high, which corresponds to a value of 3, then the overall satisfaction score would be 10 - 3 = 7, in other words, a satisfied client.

According to a study conducted by the Marketing Science Institute, clients have 10 key expectations where you should endeavour to achieve excellence (Table 7).

Table 7. Key client expectations.

Key client expectations	
Reliability	Communication
Responsiveness	Credibility
Professionalism	Security
Accessibility	Client knowledge and understanding
Courtesy	Tangible elements: appearance of the clinic, veterinary equipment, etc.

Methods for measuring satisfaction levels

Measures

- Suggestion box: easy to implement and cheap, but it is hard to obtain a representative sample.
- Send out an easy-to-complete offline and online questionnaire. In general, no more than 35 % of recipients open these emails.
- Physically gather information with an emoticons table. There are companies that hire or sell a kind of tablet especially configured to collect data and analyse the responses. They are often found in airports, bars, etc. You can obtain more than 10 responses in just 60 seconds.

The data you gather should be assessed using the NPS method explained in Chapter 5.

Action plans

Action plans creation stage

Continuing the client analysis, you must also take into account two important factors: the number of loyal clients and the return they produce. We all have clients who, for years, only visit the clinic for vaccinations and in case of emergencies, but they do not produce a high average sale. It is important to segment clients using the following matrix, so you can then apply strategies to each segment, and even opt to neglect those low-loyalty clients who represent a low return on investment (Fig. 7).

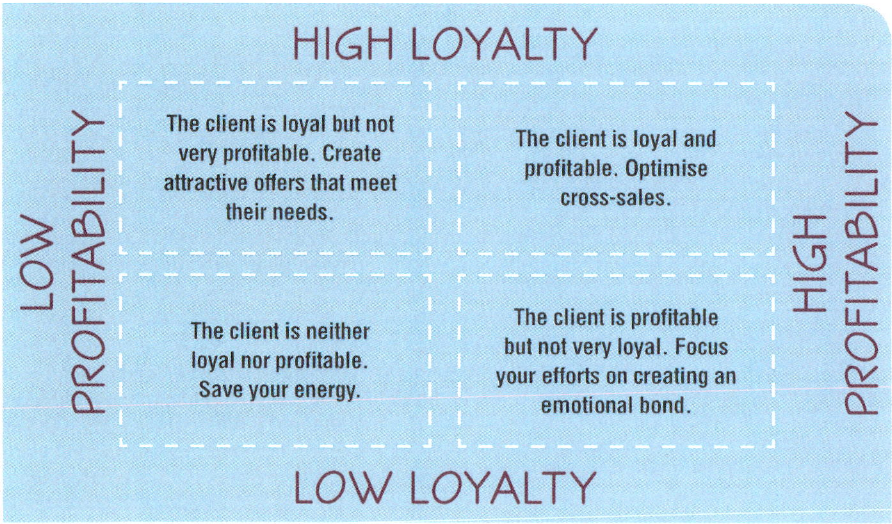
HIGH LOYALTY
LOW PROFITABILITY
The client is loyal but not very profitable. Create attractive offers that meet their needs.
The client is loyal and profitable. Optimise cross-sales.
HIGH PROFITABILITY
The client is neither loyal nor profitable. Save your energy.
The client is profitable but not very loyal. Focus your efforts on creating an emotional bond.
LOW LOYALTY

Figure 7. Method for segmenting clients.

The next step is to create some action plans with the aid of the CAME analysis and a good client segmentation based on the new matrix. These will help you schedule the order and choose the right time to implement the actions. To this end, we shall employ the matrix developed by Stephen Covey in his book *The 7 Habits of Highly Effective People*.

Remember, you must set yourself SMART goals: specific, measurable, attainable, realistic, and time-bound.

Important/Urgent	Important/Not urgent
Unimportant/Urgent	**Unimportant/Not urgent**

Improvement

Template for working on factors that create or improve the client experience

The template includes some examples to demonstrate the application of this tool, which is designed for working on SEM factors (Table 8).

Table 8. Template for working on SEM factors.

Sense	Strategy to follow	Implementation start date	End of implementation	Who will do it?	Follow-up and correction, where necessary
Smell	Create an aroma for your veterinary clinic	February	May	Peter	July. Place another diffuser in the hospitalisation area to cover visits
Taste	Offer a sweet, chocolate, etc. during payment				
Touch	Make contact by shaking hands, or placing your hand on the client's shoulder when you accompany them				
Hearing	Relaxing music in the waiting room				
Sight	Place posters of pets playing on the beach with children on the clinic's walls, reception desk, etc.				

If you like working in Excel, you can use predesigned templates, like the example that follows (Fig. 8), to develop appropriate action plans.

EXAMPLE

Hire an aromatherapy consultant for your veterinary clinic.

Task no.	Description	Person responsible	Priority status
A	**Organoleptic changes**		
1	Create aroma		
2	Change colour of rooms		
3	Emotional photos		
4			
B	**Social media management**		
1	Monthly Facebook plan		
2			
3			
4			
5			
C	**Staff training**		
1	Managerial training		
2	Vet training		
3	Auxiliary staff training		
4	Scheduling overall goals meetings		

Figure 8. Template for developing an action plan.

You must remember that, while the action plans are well defined, they must also be flexible so corrective measures can be applied whenever you believe they are necessary. Finally, always measure the return on investment (ROI) obtained from your marketing using the following equation:

ROI = (PROFIT - INVESTMENT)/INVESTMENT*

* The result will be a percentage.

Start date	Budget	Percent complete	Deadline	Days remaining
16/07/18	€5,000.00	50 %	15/08/18	180
04/09/18	€1,200.00	25 %	04/10/18	230
12/01/19	€5,000.00	30 %	11/02/19	360
18/03/18	€800.00	20 %	17/04/18	60
16/07/18	€4,000.00	75 %	15/08/18	180
16/07/18	€1,500.00	45 %	15/08/18	180
16/07/18	€5,000.00	65 %	15/08/18	180
16/07/18	€3,614.29	63 %	15/08/18	180
16/07/18	€3,600.00	68 %	15/08/18	180
16/07/18	€3,585.71	72 %	15/08/18	180
16/07/18	€3,571.43	77 %	15/08/18	180
16/07/18	€3,557.14	81 %	15/08/18	180
16/07/18	€3,542.86	86 %	15/08/18	180
16/07/18	€3,528.57	91 %	15/08/18	180
16/07/18	€3,514.29	95 %	15/08/18	180
16/07/18	€3,500.00	100 %	15/08/18	180

SUMMARY

- You must sit down and draft your own personal neuromarketing plan, bearing in mind your client segmentation and your practice's potential given the facilities, means of communication, or your staff's talent base.
- Having established this information, prioritise the actions that will have the greatest impact on your clients and profitability.
- Then you should prepare your entire team, explaining the neuromarketing plan, allocating the functions that each shall assume, and informing them about the available resources and the time frame for implementing each action.

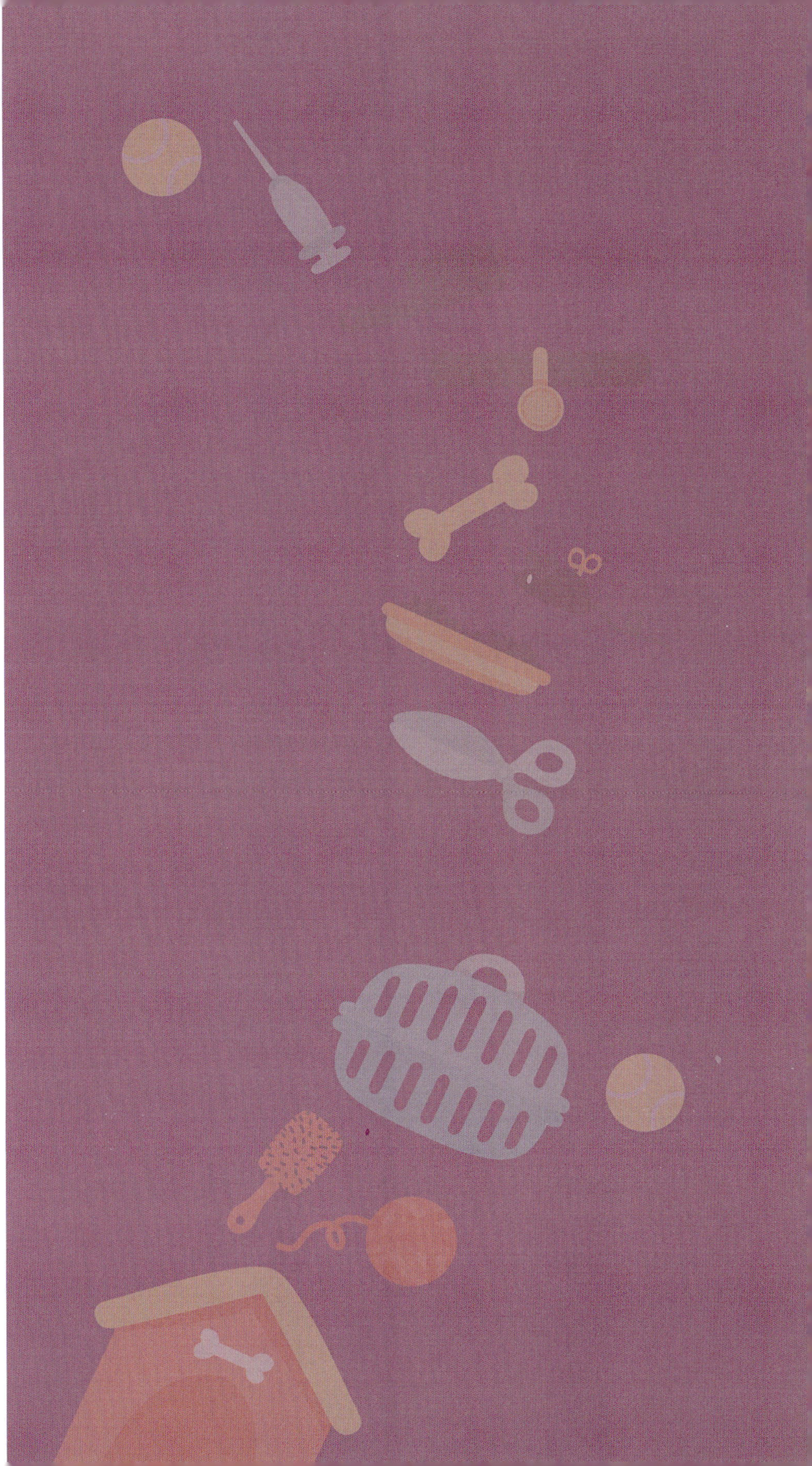

References

Adán, P. *Business to social.* SCLibro, 2015.

Albuixech, M., Alfarás, S., Atmetlla, E. et al. *Gestión Clínica Veterinaria. Marketing.* Profit Editorial, 2017.

Alcaide Casado, J. C. *Fidelización de clientes.* ESIC, 2015.

Allen, S. *Persuasión e influencia.* Create Space, 2017.

Álvarez del Blanco, R. *Neuromarketing.* Pearson educación SL, 2011.

Barbosa, P. *Speculations & Trends.* Vida Económica, 2010.

Baró, T. *La gran guía del lenguaje no verbal.* Paidós Divulgación, 2016.

Bassat, L. *El libro rojo de la publicidad.* Random House Mondadori, 2010.

Bauman, Z. *Modernidad líquida.* Edición electrónica, 2015.

Bernada, G., Osterwalder, A., Pigneur, Y., Smith, A. *Value Proposition Design.* Wiley, 2014 .

Braidot, N. *Neuromarketing.* Planeta, 2016.

Caiazo, B. *Claves del éxito en telemarketing.* Díaz de Santos, 1990.

Cialdini, R. *Pre-suasión. Un método revolucionario para influir y convencer.* Conecta, 2017.

Covey, S. R. *The 7 Habits of Highly Effective People.* Simon & Schuster, 2004.

Cram, T. *Los clientes que cuentan.* Pearson, 2003.

Dooley, R. *Brainfluence.* Ediciones Urano, 2015.

Fiol, A., Obiols, M. *Coaching para todos. Herramientas para el cambio personal y profesional.* Plataforma Editorial, 2013.

Franklin, D. *Megachange: The World in 2050.* Wiley, 2012.

García Palomo, J.P., Martínez Montes, E. *Neuromarketing. Alicia y el espejo. El otro lado del espejo.* Starbook Editorial, 2011.

Gladwell, M. *Inteligencia Intuitiva.* Penguin Random House edit, 2005.

Godin, S. *El marketing del permiso. Convertir a los extraños en amigos y a los amigos en clientes.* Ediciones Urano, 2016.

Goleman, D. *Liderazgo.* Ediciones BSA, 2013.

Goleman, D. *El cerebro y la inteligencia emocional.* SA Ediciones B, 2016.

González de la Hoz, M. *Experiencia de cliente.* LID Editorial Empresarial, 2015.

Goodman, J. A. *Atención estratégica al cliente.* Pluma digital Ediciones, 2014.

Jantsc, J. *Activa el boca-oreja.* Empresa Activa, 2011.

KAHNEMAN, D. *Thinking, Fast and Slow.* Farrar, Straus and Giroux, 2011.
KAWASAKY, G. *El arte de cautivar.* Planeta, 2011.
KIMSEY-HOUSE, H. ET AL. *Coaching Co-Activ.* Ediciones Paidós, 2014.
KLARIC, J. *Véndele a la mente no a la gente.* División Editorial, 2014.
KOCH, R. *El principio 80/20.* Espasa, 2009.
LARA COCA, M. *Aprende Copywriting en 2 horas.* Ediciones PR, 2015.
LINDSTROM, M. BUYOLOGY. Verdades y mentiras de por qué compramos. Gestión 2000. Grupo Planeta, 2010.
LINDSTROM, M. *Así se manipula al consumidor.* Grupo Planeta, 2011.
MALFITANO, O. *Neurociencias en ciencias económicas.* Alta Gerencia, 2014.
MEJÍA LLANO, J.C. *La guía avanzada del community manager.* Anaya, 2015.
MORENO MOLINA, M. *El gran libro del community manager.* Planeta, 2014.
MORIN, C., RENVOISÉ, P. Neuromarketing. *El Nervio de la venta.* Editorial UOC, 2006. Reedición 2016.
PARISER, E. *El filtro burbuja. Cómo la red decide lo que leemos y lo que pensamos.* Editorial Taurus, 2017.
PÉREZ ORTEGA, A. *Marca personal para dummies.* Planeta, 2014.
PETERS, T., AUSTIN, N. *A Passion for Excellence: The Leadership Difference.* Grand Central Publishing, 1989.
RAMÓN-CORTÉS, F., GALOFRE, A. *Relaciones que funcionan. Cómo entenderte hasta con tu peor enemigo.* Conecta, 2015.
RUIS PARDO, J. *Neuropymes.* Pirámide editorial, 2013.
SINEK, S. *La clave es el porqué.* Península, 2013.
TRACY, B. *El arte de cerrar la venta.* Grupo Nelson, 2007.
VALERA, M.A. *Planes de salud.* Servet, 2017.
VILLEGAS SAURÍ, S. *Marketingdencias.* Planeta, 2014.
ZIGLAR, Z. *Ventas 101.* Grupo Nelson, 2012.

www.argosportalveterinaria.com
www.estudiosveterinarios.com
www.mascotasyplanes.com

Published by Servet editorial - Grupo Asís Biomedia S.L.